I0023504

OLYMPIC LIFTING

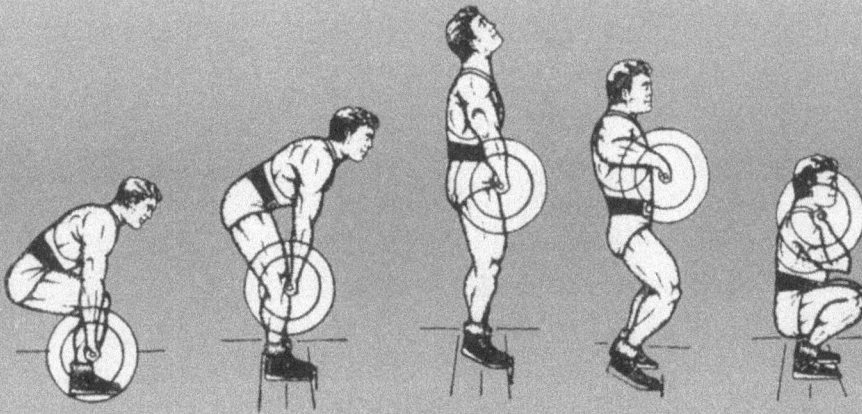

A TRAINING MANUAL

CARL MILLER

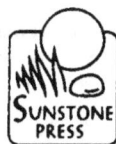

SUNSTONE
PRESS

SANTA FE

© 2018 by Carl Miller
All Rights Reserved
No part of this book may be reproduced in any form or by any electronic or mechanical means including
information storage and retrieval systems without permission in writing from the publisher,
except by a reviewer who may quote brief passages in a review.

Sunstone books may be purchased for educational, business, or sales promotional use.
For information please write: Special Markets Department, Sunstone Press,
P.O. Box 2321, Santa Fe, New Mexico 87504-2321.

Cover design › Vicki Ahl
Printed on acid-free paper
☉

Library of Congress Cataloging-in-Publication Data

On File

ISBN: 978-1-63293-218-1

SUNSTONE PRESS IS COMMITTED TO MINIMIZING OUR ENVIRONMENTAL IMPACT ON THE PLANET. THE PAPER USED IN THIS BOOK IS
FROM RESPONSIBLY MANAGED FORESTS. OUR PRINTER HAS RECEIVED CHAIN OF CUSTODY (COC) CERTIFICATION FROM: THE FOREST
STEWARDSHIP COUNCIL™ (FSC®), PROGRAMME FOR THE ENDORSEMENT OF FOREST CERTIFICATION™ (PEFC™), AND THE SUSTAINABLE
FORESTRY INITIATIVE® (SFI®). THE FSC® COUNCIL IS A NON-PROFIT ORGANIZATION, PROMOTING THE ENVIRONMENTALLY
APPROPRIATE, SOCIALLY BENEFICIAL AND ECONOMICALLY VIABLE MANAGEMENT OF THE WORLD'S FORESTS. FSC® CERTIFICATION IS
RECOGNIZED INTERNATIONALLY AS A RIGOROUS ENVIRONMENTAL AND SOCIAL STANDARD FOR RESPONSIBLE FOREST MANAGEMENT.

WWW.SUNSTONEPRESS.COM
SUNSTONE PRESS / POST OFFICE BOX 2321 / SANTA FE, NM 87504-2321 /USA
(505) 988-4418 / ORDERS ONLY (800) 243-5644 / FAX (505) 988-1025

Dedicated to Bob Crist

National Weightlifting Chairman

1971 to 1975

Contents

Preface

WHY THESE WRITINGS HAVE BEEN ASSEMBLED

These writings have been assembled in order to bring them into relative continuity and to show how they blend into each other in the total approach needed for a successful weightlifting program. In addition, writings from 1976 are included here, material which was not presented at clinics because of the great reduction in number of clinics held. These are valuable in themselves and are also important in how they fit into the total approach to lifting.

I would like to suggest that the reader first read these writings looking for organized categories, then see how the details fit in. My main concern was to bring order to the myriad of weightlifting knowledge contained in these articles.

The Bulgaria articles and the Marseille-Moscow articles should not be viewed as the Bulgarian System or the French System or the Russian System. These were reports written after I returned from these places, hence these titles. Therefore, these reports are not based on any pure national system but are my own attempts to organize vast amounts of material at certain periods of my tenure as National Coaching Coordinator.

Each reader should adapt the material to his own stage of development in weightlifting. Many of the training routines, for example, are organized as to Class Categories. If a lifter ranks in Class II and the Class II training routines are too hard, he should feel free to drop down to the Class III or even the Class IV training routines. In any writings, broad general categories must be viewed with individual flexibility. These categories are meant to give meaningful structure and organization, without which chaos results, but to adhere to them rigidly is certainly a mistake. The athlete functions best within organized knowledge of the whole picture. When viewed this way, flexibility adds to his performance.

A great number of coaches and athletes from other sports have read these writings and have said how well organized they are and how easy they are to follow. These are coaches and athletes who have poured over materials in their own respective sports about which so much has been written. Weightlifting is in its infancy as far as the organizing and writing down of knowledge. Relatively little has been written when compared to other sports. Hopefully, this compiling of my writings as National Coaching Coordinator will stimulate more knowledge to be organized and put into writing because this material should be considered only a beginning. It is up to date and extremely useful, but still only a beginning.

C.M.

SECTION I

SELECTION OF WEIGHTLIFTERS

Specifics of Selecting Top Weightlifters - Bulgaria #2

In this, the second report on my trip to Bulgaria, I want to talk about a process for selecting top weightlifters. This was not only discussed extensively at the conference but it is also very applicable to us in the United States. We are starting to get quantities of young lifters into our programs, and I think we realize we also have to be very cognizant of quality. While it is our aim to interest many boys in our program so as to form a wide base and a healthier America, we also have to get the quality so we can have the material that will be able to do well in international competition.

Selection really cannot be overemphasized because it is at this stage that we hope to interest a person who may be with us for years. Does he really possess the physical qualities that it takes to be a top lifter? If we do not find out in the beginning, much of our work to encourage lifters of international caliber will become wasted on lifters who just were not meant to have that amount of time spent on them. It is much more productive to choose right from the start somebody who does have potential in our sport. However, let us not deceive ourselves; a selection process is not foolproof. There will still be many disappointments, many casualties, but a process such as the one that has been used by the Bulgarians can be a great success. It is their selection of talent that I believe is one of the most important keys to their success. Their selection process has not been duplicated in other countries. Even the Russians say they have not done what the Bulgarians have done in selection.

In selecting weightlifters we want to choose young men who have a real aptitude for lifting. There are some very good tests which are highly correlated with lifting ability. While the Bulgarians use many tests, I believe that these can and should be simplified for our purposes. Many of the tests overlap; that is to say, some tests are so inclusive that it is not to any advantage to have two tests when one will do the job. Statistical analysis of these tests prove this; it is not just my opinion, rather it is a fact. Also, our liaison with the physical education departments of our junior high schools, high schools and other places where youth engage in sports (e.g. recreation departments, YMCAs, Boys Clubs) is not professionally set up as it is in Bulgaria. What we want are meaningful tests that the physical education instructor or recreation director is familiar with and uses in his program or can easily use if asked.

The first test is the standing broad jump. This measures an athlete's leg, hip and back power which is so important to a lifter. The coordination of these muscles in the standing broad jump is also similar to lifting. The test is important because it measures something basic, namely explosiveness, and you either have this or you don't in these muscle groups. Below is how to administer the test and score it.

Warm-up Activities Warm-up activities should consist of alternating jogging, running for 30 yards, and walking for a period of three or four minutes, followed by shadow rope skipping, triple jumping (hop, step and jump), hopping, and leaping for three or four minutes. The jumping test should follow as soon as the pupil has resumed normal breathing.

Test Event The pupil stands with feet several inches apart and with toes just back of the takeoff line or front edge of the takeoff board or mark. The takeoff is made from both feet, and the pupil jumps forward as far as possible, landing on both feet. Free swinging of the arms and bending of the knees is permissable, but during this action of arms and legs the feet must not leave the board or takeoff line until the jump is made.

Rules 1. Three fair trials shall be allowed and the best of the three recorded.
2. The pupil's performance is recorded in inches to the nearest inch.
3. Measure from the takeoff line to the heel or any part of the body that touches the surface nearest the takeoff line.

PERCENTILE SCORES FOR THE STANDING BROAD JUMP
ACCORDING TO AGE AND LENGTH OF JUMP AS MEASURED IN INCHES

Percentile score	Age 10	Age 11	Age 12	Age 13	Age 14	Age 15	Age 16	Age 17	Age 18	Age 19
95	70	74	80	86	94	98	100	103	103	105
90	68	72	76	83	91	94	95	98	99	101
85	65	70	74	80	89	92	93	97	97	99
80	65	68	72	79	87	90	92	95	96	98
75	64	66	71	76	85	89	90	92	94	96
70	63	64	70	75	85	87	89	91	92	94
65	63	63	70	74	83	86	88	89	91	93
60	62	63	68	73	82	85	87	88	90	92
55	62	62	67	72	80	84	86	87	89	91
50	61	61	66	71	79	83	85	86	88	89
45	59	60	66	70	78	82	84	85	87	88
40	56	59	65	69	76	80	82	85	86	87
35	55	58	64	68	75	79	81	84	85	86
30	53	56	63	67	73	78	79	82	83	85
25	51	55	62	66	72	76	77	80	82	84
20	48	54	60	65	70	76	74	78	80	82
15	48	52	59	62	68	73	72	76	79	81
10	47	48	55	60	65	71	70	73	76	79
5	43	48	50	56	62	67	66	68	72	76

The second test is the 50 yard dash. This measures many of the same things that the standing broad jump measures but they are not correlated highly enough for either to be used as a sole test for these things. Maybe it comes down to neuromotor specificity. The work of the Bulgarians shows that good lifters do very well on both the standing broad jump and the 50 yard dash, while not-so-good lifters may show up good on one but not the other.

Warm-up Activities Warm-up activities should consist of a normal walking pace to a fast walk, to a jog for 200 to 300 yards; a slow jogging then to a fast sprinting for 300 yards.

Facilities and Equipment a 70 yard straight running surface with starting and finishing lines 50 yards apart, a 20 yard space beyond the finish line, and a stop watch

Test Event The runner takes his position behind the starting line. Either a standing or a crouch start may be used. The crouch start is recommended only for pupils who have had instruction and practice in this technique. The starter takes a position at the starting line and uses these commands: "get on your mark" - preparatory command to alert all runners, "set" - spoken when all runners indicate they are ready by being motionless and looking directly down the track, and "go" - spoken by the starter approximately two seconds after the "set" command. The word

9

"go" should be accompanied by a downward sweep of the starter's arm as a signal to the timer standing at the finish line to start the stop watch.

Rules
1. Only one trial may be given.
2. A reasonable warm-up should precede the test.
3. The score is the time elapsed between the starting signal and the moment the runner crosses the finish line.
4. Scoring shall be recorded in seconds and tenths of seconds.

PERCENTILE SCORES FOR THE 50 YARD DASH
ACCORDING TO AGE AND DURATION OF RUN AS MEASURED IN SECONDS

Percentile score	Age 10	Age 11	Age 12	Age 13	Age 14	Age 15	Age 16	Age 17	Age 18	Age 19+
95	7.0	7.0	6.8	6.7	6.4	6.3	6.1	6.2	6.0	5.9
90	7.4	7.3	7.1	6.9	6.5	6.4	6.2	6.3	6.3	6.0
85	7.5	7.4	7.3	7.0	6.6	6.5	6.3	6.4	6.3	6.2
80	7.8	7.4	7.4	7.1	6.7	6.6	6.4	6.5	6.3	6.3
75	7.9	7.5	7.5	7.2	6.8	6.7	6.5	6.5	6.4	6.3
70	8.0	7.6	7.6	7.2	6.9	6.8	6.6	6.6	6.5	6.4
65	8.1	7.8	7.7	7.3	7.0	6.9	6.6	6.6	6.6	6.5
60	8.2	8.0	7.8	7.4	7.1	6.9	6.7	6.7	6.6	6.6
55	8.3	8.1	7.9	7.5	7.1	7.0	6.8	6.7	6.7	6.7
50	8.4	8.2	7.9	7.6	7.2	7.0	6.8	6.8	6.8	6.7
45	8.4	8.3	8.0	7.6	7.3	7.1	6.9	6.8	6.9	6.8
40	8.5	8.4	8.1	7.7	7.4	7.2	7.0	7.0	6.9	6.9
35	8.6	8.4	8.2	7.8	7.4	7.2	7.1	7.0	7.0	7.0
30	8.8	8.5	8.4	8.0	7.5	7.3	7.1	7.1	6.9	7.0
25	8.9	8.6	8.5	8.1	7.6	7.4	7.2	7.1	7.0	7.1
20	9.1	8.9	8.6	8.2	7.8	7.5	7.3	7.2	7.0	7.1
15	9.3	9.1	8.8	8.3	7.9	7.6	7.4	7.4	7.1	7.2
10	9.4	9.3	9.0	8.5	8.2	7.6	7.6	7.8	7.2	7.2
5	9.7	9.6	9.4	8.8	8.6	8.0	8.0	7.9	7.6	7.4

The third test is the chin-up. While this would not seem to be a good test since the pulling is in a different direction than that in lifting, it has been highly correlated with good lifting ability in Europe and is used to select lifters. I believe that the main thing being tested is the strength of the traps. Yes, the arms do bend and are used as are the lats, but the traps play both an active and a stabilizing part and, therefore, this could be the reason the test relates so well to lifting successfully.

Warm-up Activities   The warm-up activities should consist of a three or four minute period of jogging, running and walking. Such exercises as jumping jacks, windmill, arm circling, and climbing a vertical pole or rope climb should be done. After a three minute rest the test should be administered while the pupil is still warm.

Facilities and Equipment   a metal chinning bar

Test Event   The bar should be at a height that will permit the pupil to hand so that his arms and legs are fully extended a few inches above the ground. He should grasp the bar with a forward grip (back of hands to face). He then raises his body by his arms until his chin is above the bar, and then he lowers his body to a full hang as in the starting position.

Rules   1. Only one trial shall be allowed, unless for some reason the teacher

10

believes that the pupil has not had a fair opportunity.
2. The body must not swing during the execution of the movement. The pull must in no way be a snap movement.
3. The knees must not be raised, and kicking of the legs is not permitted.
4. One complete pull-up is counted each time the pupil places his chin above the bar.

PERCENTILE SCORES FOR THE PULL-UP
ACCORDING TO AGE AND NUMBER OF PULL-UPS PERFORMED

Percentile score	Age 10	Age 11	Age 12	Age 13	Age 14	Age 15	Age 16	Age 17	Age 18	Age 19+
95	9	7	9	11	14	15	17	19	18	20
90	7	6	8	10	12	13	15	16	16	17
85	6	5	7	9	11	12	13	15	14	16
80	6	5	6	8	10	11	12	14	15	15
75	4	4	6	7	9	10	12	12	12	14
70	4	4	5	6	8	9	10	12	12	13
65	4	3	4	6	7	9	10	11	11	13
60	3	3	4	5	7	8	10	10	11	12
55	2	3	3	5	6	8	9	10	10	11
50	2	2	2	4	6	7	9	9	10	11
45	2	2	2	4	5	6	8	8	9	10
40	2	2	2	3	5	6	8	8	9	9
35	1	1	2	3	4	5	7	7	8	9
30	1	1	1	2	4	5	6	6	8	8
25	0	1	0	2	3	4	6	6	7	7
20	0	0	0	2	3	3	5	5	6	7
15	0	0	0	2	2	3	3	4	5	6
10	0	0	0	1	2	2	2	3	3	5
5	0	0	0	0	0	2	0	2	2	3

The fourth test is to have the prospective lifter squat down with his feet shoulder distance apart and see if he can sit straight with his feet flat on the floor, his rear end ahead of his heels. This tests ankle flexibility. While this flexibility can develop to some extent, it is a tremendous asset to a lifter to have flexible ankles from the beginning. All the pulling positions plus the bottom and jerking positions revolve around this joint which is not the easiest in the body to develop as far as flexibility is concerned.

The fifth test, the only subjective one, is how does the athlete react competitively in sports which are somewhat related to lifting. These would be sports that are taught in physical education or recreational programs and which an instructor would have observed. They are sports which are somewhat explosive in nature and take concentration before attempting. These are also sports which give an athlete time to think between performances. Does it seem that the athlete can concentrate and get the most out of himself? Is he cool under pressure? Does he rise to the occasion or does he melt and fall apart? Some people with time between athletic performances improve, others do not. A positive performance can be taught but it is difficult. It is much better to have an athlete who already has this quality. Some of the activities and sports which we are talking about are: shot put, pole vault, javelin, high jump, broad jump, gymnastics and wrestling.

These tests are very inclusive. They cannot, naturally, give you a blueprint of a champion. Their usefulness is in their inclusiveness. In other words, when you give the tests, they tell you a lot about whether an athlete would be a candidate to be a good lifter. A score on each test of the 80th percentile or better is indicative of a good prospect. A high subjective score on the fifth test, the psychological aspect by an athlete's PE teacher, coach or recreational supervisor, should be greatly valued. There are many physically gifted athletes who are a waste of time simply because they have not "got it" psychologically to compete. That is not to say such an athlete is less of a person, but that he is not a suitable prospect for the international platform.

One further comment on the fourth test, the ankle flexibility test, is that this is something the prospective lifter either passes or fails. Some who take this test will be tight in the ankles from lack of conditioning; these can be pushed into the desired position. If you can push the prospect into a squat with his feet shoulder distance apart, sitting straight with his feet flat on the floor with his rear end ahead of his heels, then he does have ample ankle flexibility. This "positioning" can be done by pushing down and back on the shoulders with one hand and pushing the hips down and forward with the other.

So here is a tool for selection. I urge our coaches and administrators to use it. Get to know at least one physical education teacher or recreation director in your area, more than one if you have time. Cultivate a rapport with him. Ask him if he has any athletes who have scored well in the above areas. Ask him if they are available. Some, naturally, will be out for other sports, but there will be many who are not. We have not and the majority of the world has not begun to tap the potential fine weightlifters. That is why the records are going to continue to go up and why it is important that we be first to tap this talent.

SECTION II

STYLE

1

Double Knee Bend

The double knee bend is a summation of largely straight forces from the floor to the top of the pull. Let us go through some of the highlights which make it so.

The lifter should make as fast a start as possible with the leverage at hand. The increasing of the speed should take place all along the pull as optimum points of leverage are reached and succeeding speed built on what went before. This is different from deliberately pulling slow off the floor. The lifter should make use of every leverage point. He should not yank the bar in an effort to get speed, and he should not break good body position. In other words, the lifter should go as fast as the leverage at hand will permit with good body position.

The weight of the body is centered on the front part of the instep when starting the pull. This does not mean he is on his toes as the whole foot is in contact with the floor. It means that when pressure is exerted by the feet, the center seems to be at the front part of the instep. Then the weight of the body is transferred back as the bar is lifted to the knees. Also, as the bar is lifted from the floor the hips are kept in. They do not shoot back. They go up vertically because the knees are straightening. As the knees straighten the bar is brought slightly back about two inches from its initial position which was over the metatarsals. The angle of the back is constant from the floor to the knees.

As the bar comes past the knees, the weight of the body is at the furthest point back. It has come from the balls of the feet (front part of the instep) back to the middle of the feet. From this position the weight must return to the balls of the feet again. This is very important. Some lifters get into the correct position for the second pull but their weight is still centered on the middle of the feet, not on the balls of the feet. So then they are off balance and they pull in a rotation instead of straight up.

With the bar past the knees, the bar having been brought back about two inches and the bodyweight coming forward, the knees bend (they are bending a second time; they were bent to start with when the bar was pulled off the floor) and the hips come down and forward, and the back comes up. The bending of the knees causes the down and forward action. The lifter is becoming more erect as the back rises, with the bodyweight transferring to the balls of the feet, the whole foot in contact with the floor. This has been described as a scooping action. It is in this manner that the lifter gets his body into the best possible pulling position. If this is not done right, what commonly happens is the hips come down and forward but the bodyweight stays back. This results later in a rotation. Then when the lifter does his second pull, there is a continuation of this rotation and a rotary force is added onto the preceding straight forces so that they do not add up to as much resulting force as would the addition of straight forces. Thus the lifter does not get the maximum pull, and many times the bar is lost behind and he jumps back.

When the body is in the best pulling position, the second pull causes great acceleration of the bar. The preceding scooping action is done faster than the first pull but the main acceleration comes from the second pull. (It should be emphasized that the whole pulling action from the floor to overhead is one smooth pull with increasing acceleration.) This second pull is started by accelerating the scooping action of the legs and hips. As these big muscles accelerate the bar, the extension of the back then blends in (not before). This results in a continuation of the upward motion which is further continued by the later blending in of the elevation of the shoulders. The end of the pull results in the lifter up on his toes, body fully elongated (extended), shoulders shrugged. Maximum height with maximum force has been implemented to the bar.

The second pull can be thought of as a pushing away from the platform or jumping with a weight in the hands. When done right, it gives the impression of a sudden elongation or lengthening of the body. This is because the motion takes off straight up.

These are some of the highlights of the pull. Let me briefly review them in outline form.

1. The lifter starts from the floor as fast as possible with the leverage at hand.

2. The angle of the back is constant from the floor to the knees.

3. The bodyweight starts off on the front part of the instep (balls of feet) when the bar is pulled from the floor, shifts to the middle of the feet when the bar is at the knees, then back to the balls of the feet for the second pull, the whole foot being in contact with the floor throughout.

4. During the whole pull, the hips must not go back.

5. The lifter is on the balls of his feet with the whole foot in contact with the floor for the start of the second pull.

6. From nearly a straight position at the end of the first pull, the knees go into a bent position again during the scoop to the start of the second pull. This scoop is done by the hips coming down and forward and the back rising up.

7. The second pull is started by an acceleration of the scooping action as the weight of the body is transferred to the balls of the feet, the whole foot being in contact with the floor. Here the legs and hips accelerate in an upward motion. The extension of the back blends in after the action of the legs and hips.

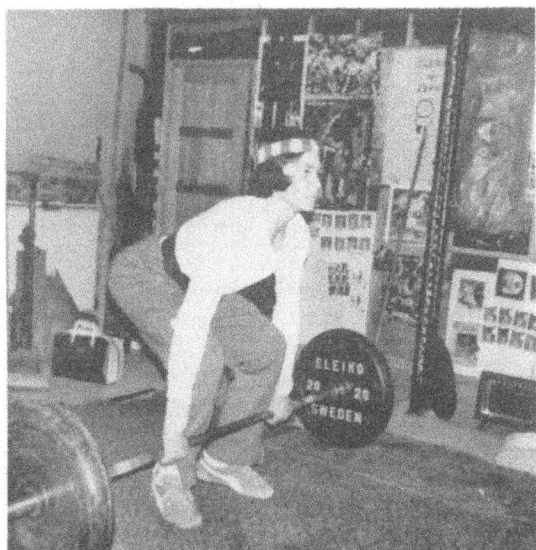

1. The bodyweight is on the front part of the instep (balls of the feet).

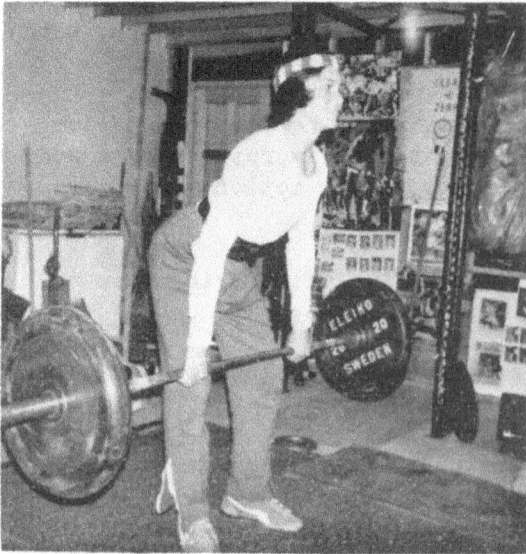

2. To get the bar to knee height the
   knees have straightened and the hips
   have come up but not back. The shoulders have gone out front. The back
   angle from the floor to here has remained constant. The bodyweight has
   shifted backward toward the middle of
   the feet.

3. The lifter has scooped into the bar.
   This is done by bending the knees,
   the hips come forward and down, the
   bodyweight shifts from the middle of
   the feet to the balls of the feet,
   and the whole foot stays in contact
   with the floor. The back has gone
   up. This is the strongest position
   from which to pull. From here all
   motion is directed up. The scoop
   carries into this. It is a lift up.

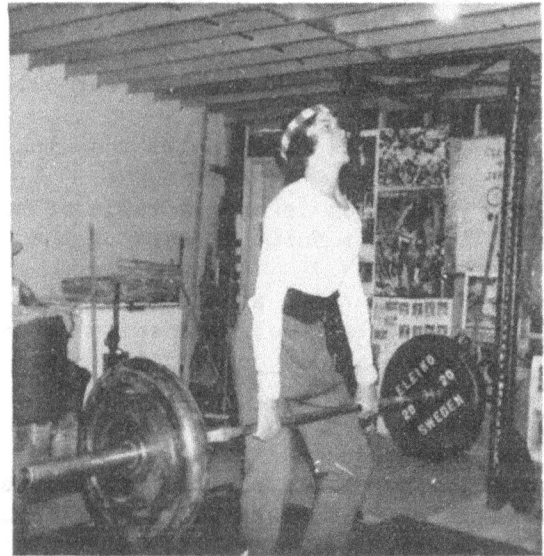

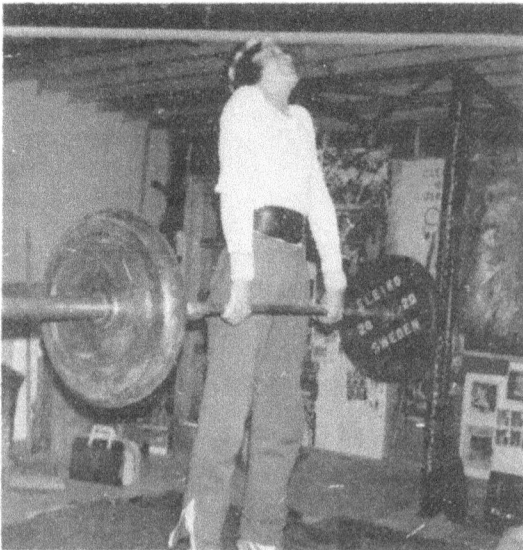

4. From the position in picture #3, the
   lifter has continued the scoop by
   straightening his legs and hips and
   then (not before) his back. The
   shoulders have elevated. This is a
   fully elongated position; note the
   straightened knees and lifter on his
   toes. A summation of straight forces
   has caused this.

2

Double Knee Bend - A Way to Learn It

When the end of the Olympic lifting year arrives for lifters, they are relaxing a bit and looking forward to the next lifting season. This is a good time to plan a cycling routine for the next lifting season. A cycling routine will take the pressure off when the lifter starts lifting again. This would also be a good time to learn thoroughly the pull popularly known as the double knee bend. Here are six exercises in the proper sequence to learn the pull.

Exercise #1 - Shrug: From the second pull position from the boxes or bar at the crotch, straighten the legs and hips, then blend in the back extension, and then shrug the shoulders straight up. Hold the top shrugged position on the toes for 3 seconds. If you do it right, you can keep your balance. If coordination is not good, you will fall forward or backward - usually backward. The head should be kept level, not thrown back; higher elevation of the shoulders can be gotten this way. The head going back will throw your balance to the rear, and the shoulders will not elevate high and will probably go back instead of up. Do three singles in four to five sets.

Exercise #2 - Clean or Snatch from Second Pull Position: When you have learned the sequence of legs, hips, back and shoulder shrug, you will consistently maintain this balanced shrugged position. Next you should snatch or clean from the second pull position from blocks or from the bar at the crotch. Use about 40-50% of your next projected goal to start with. Do three singles, four to five sets. If this exercise is too difficult, then go back to exercise #1. What is wanted is a pull that goes straight up and not back. Check to see that the final elevation of the shoulders is straight up and is complete.

In going through exercises #3,4,5 and 6 always use exercises #1 and #2 first. In the progression from exercise #3 through #6 use 70-80% of your next projected goal as a guide to when to move on to the next exercise. This will be a relatively light weight since 70-80% of your next peaking goal will be light because this is the beginning of your year of cycling. When exercise #5 is reached, do #5a and #5b at the same time. With the coordination the lifter will have picked up by this time he is at a comfortable enough stage to work the scoop both from the floor and from the knees. This leads the lifter to a natural overlap of stages that blend the coordination into one beautiful pull. These exercises are done with the clean and the snatch grip. Work each grip twice a week, either in separate sessions, making a total of four very short workouts per week, or together making two workouts per week. If you do the latter, start one time with the snatch grip, the next time with the clean grip.

Exercise #3 - Knee Scoop: From the blocks at knee height or in a power rack, assume the position attained after the Olympic dead lift. Scoop by letting the knees rebend, hips go down and forward, bodyweight goes forward onto the balls of the feet with the whole foot in contact with the floor, and the back comes up. The position reached is the second pull position with the bodyweight on the balls of the feet, whole foot in contact with the floor, and the back 15-25 degrees from the vertical, head is level and knees are rebent. It is very important to stop here; this is how the lifter learns where the second pull begins. The hardest aspect will be coordinating the action of the knees, hips, bodyweight, feet and back. A scooping action best describes it. The raising of the back is slower than the rebending of the knees and the bodyweight going onto the balls of the feet. The two common mistakes are the back coming up too soon and the back being too vertical so that the bodyweight never gets transferred back from the middle of the feet to the balls of the feet, and a rotation backwards results. Do three singles, four to five sets.

Exercise #4 - Olympic Dead Lift to Knees: With the back angle held constant, pull the weight off the floor slowly to the knees. The knees almost straighten, the hips go up vertically, not back, and the bodyweight goes from the balls of the feet to the middle of the feet. Concentrate all the time on: (1) keeping the back angle constant, (2) knees almost straightening, (3) rear end going up vertically, not back, (4) shoulders laying out in front of the bar and (5) bodyweight going from balls of feet to middle of feet. Do three singles, four to five sets.

Exercise #5a - Combined Olympic Dead Lift and Scoop: This is probably the most difficult exercise because you must coordinate the bar coming past the knees. Again, remember you must stop after the scoop with the weight forward on the balls of the feet, whole foot in contact with the floor and the back angle at 15-25 degrees from the vertical with knees bent, head level. Do three singles, four to five sets.

Exercise #5b - Combined Scoop with Shrug: From knee height off boxes or rack assume position already described when bar is at knees in exercise #4. Go through the positions of scoop and shrug as already described. Do not forget to stay on your toes for three seconds. Do three singles, four to five sets.

Exercise #6 - Olympic Dead Lift, Scoop and Shrug (High Pull with Straight Arms): This is the moment of truth. If every stage has been learned correctly, the bar should be pulled in a straight line with straight force adding on top of straight force for a maximum possible force. When doing this exercise for the first few times, go slowly and feel the movements you are going through. End up on your toes and stay there for three seconds. As you feel confident in what you are doing, go slowly off the floor, then the scoop should be a little faster, and finally the second pull should really accelerate with the shoulder elevation straight up. As form is more consistent, eliminate staying on the toes for three seconds. Do three singles, four to five sets.

Exercise #1 - Shrug

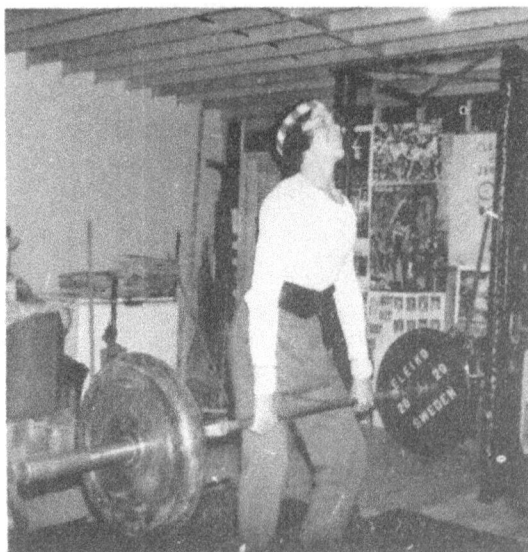
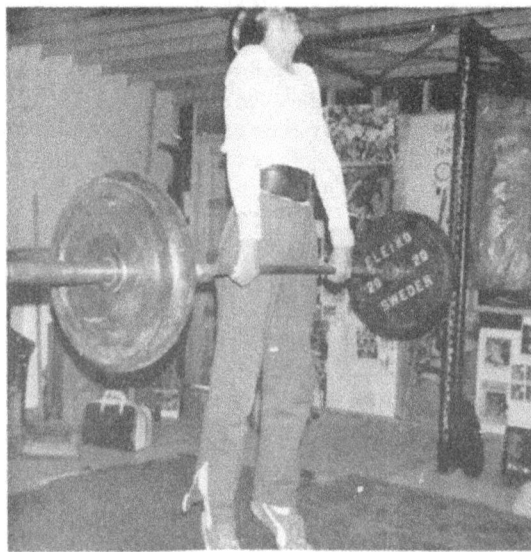

18

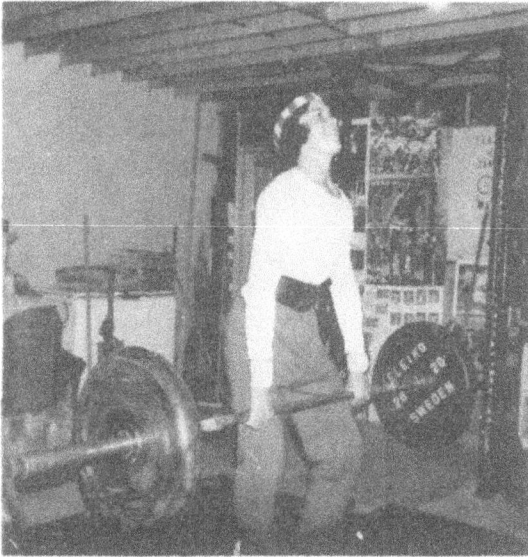

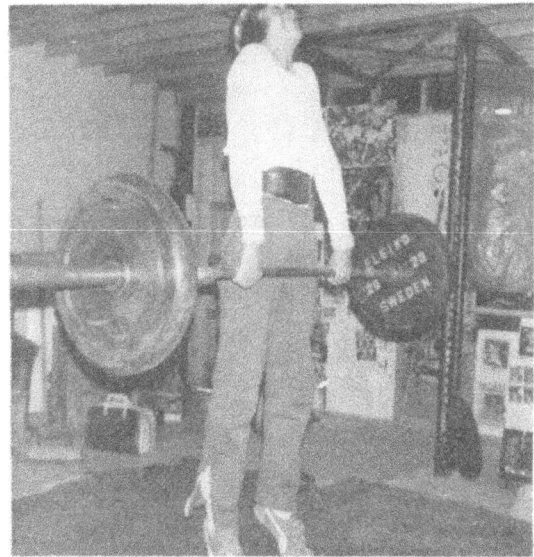

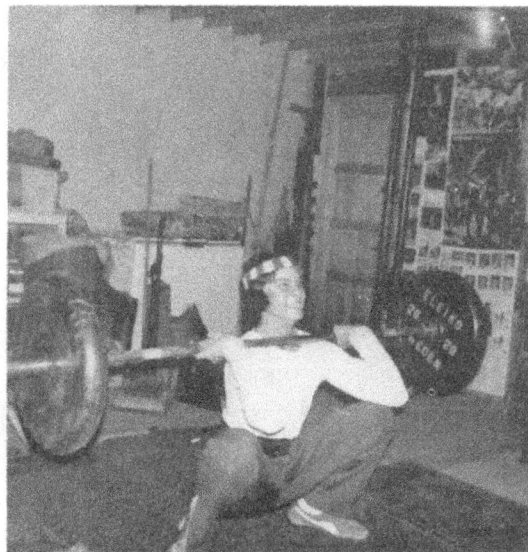

Exercise #2 - Clean or Snatch from Second Pull Position

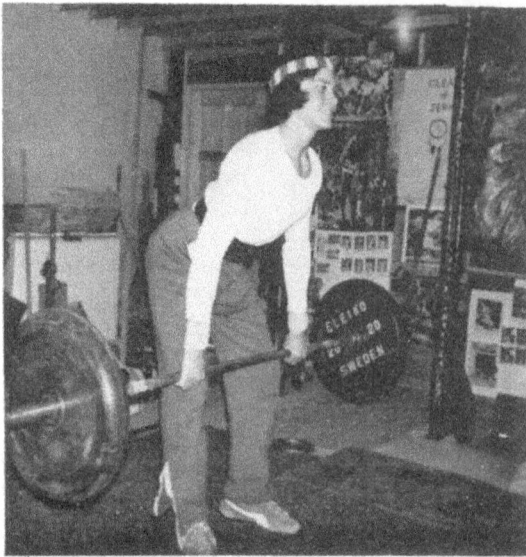
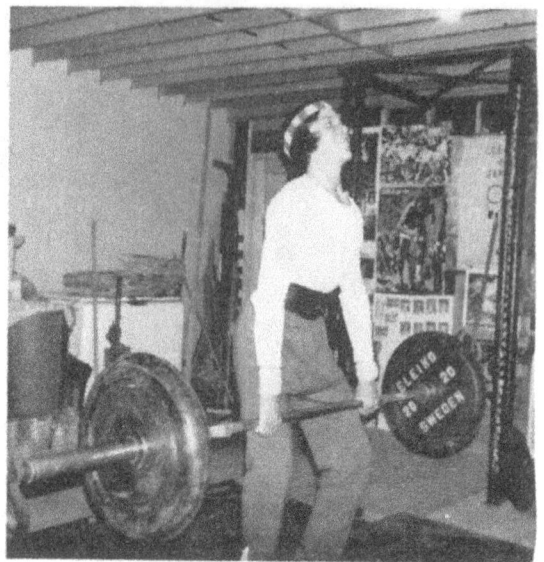

Exercise #3 - Knee Scoop

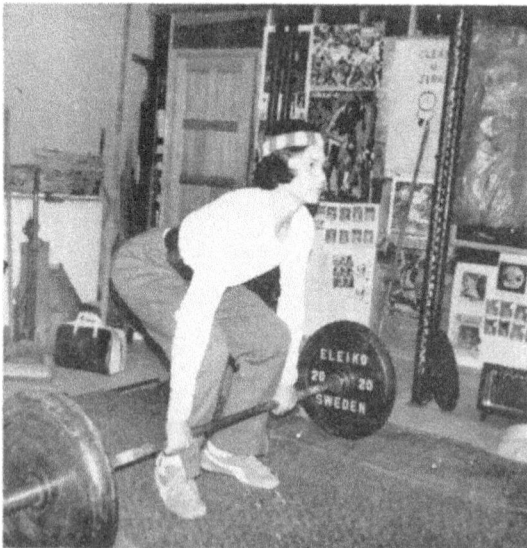
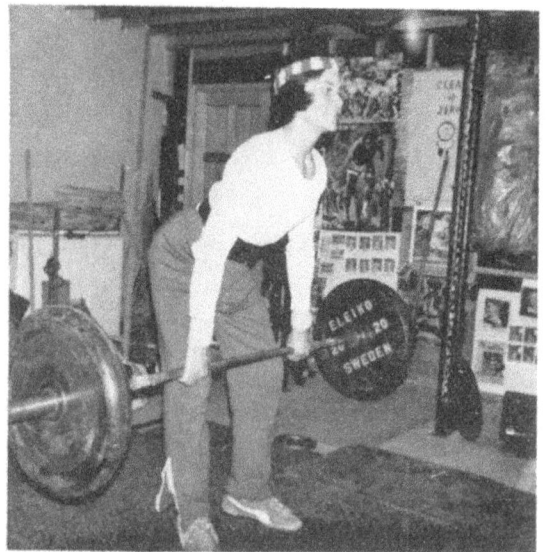

Exercise #4 - Olympic Dead Lift to Knees

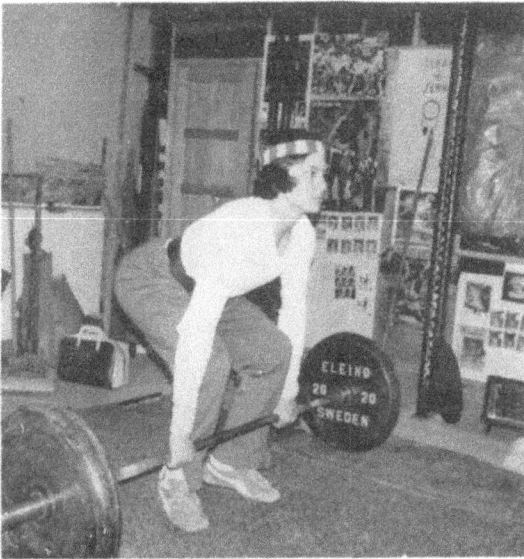

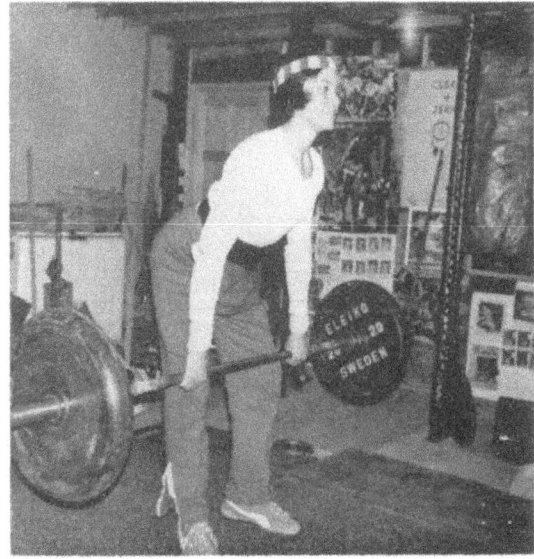

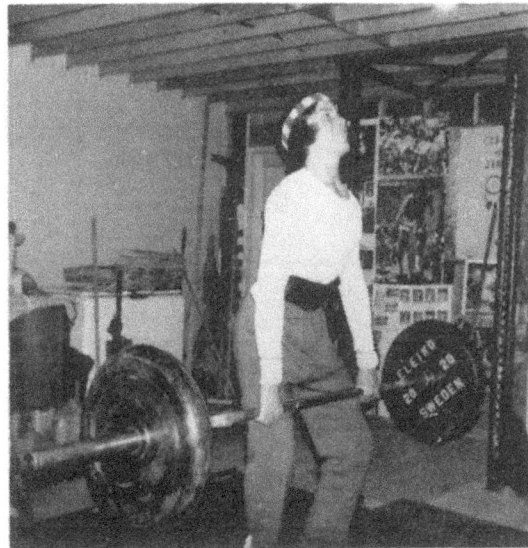

Exercise #5a - Combined Olympic Dead Lift and Scoop

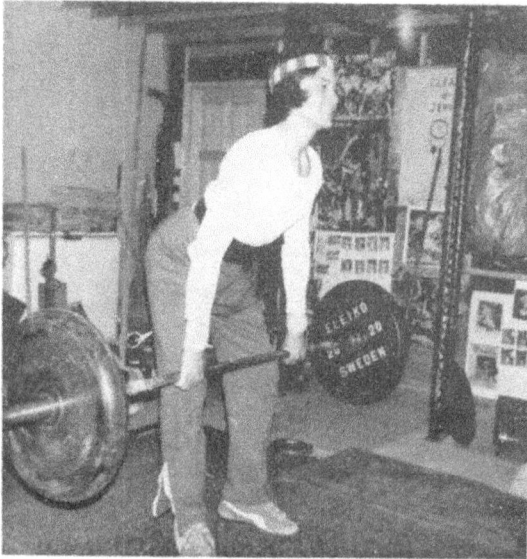

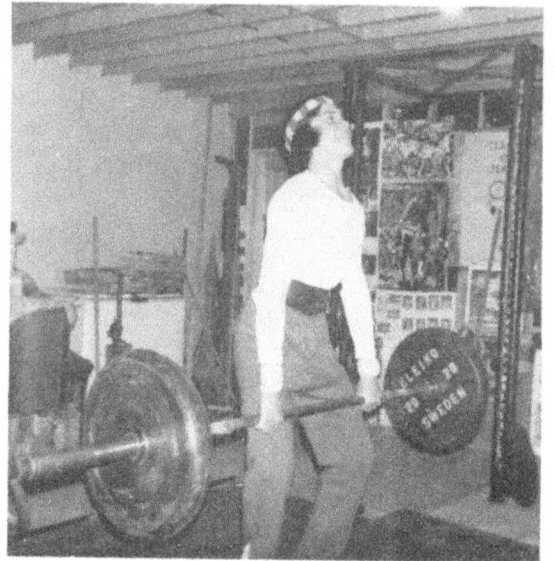

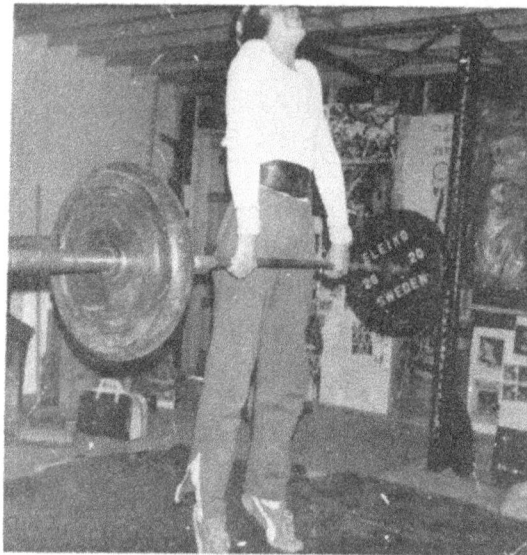

Exercise #5b - Combined Scoop with Shrug

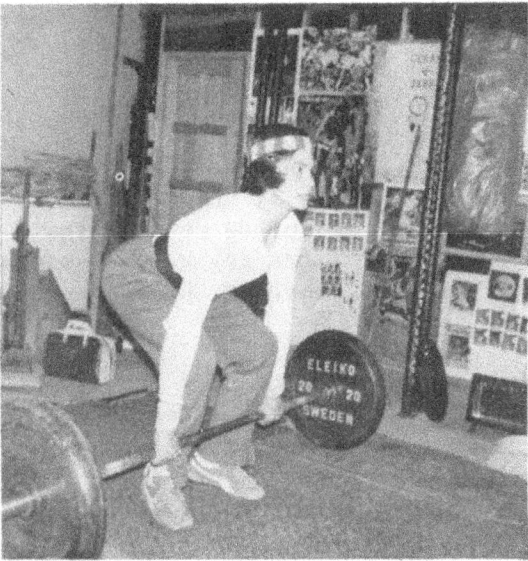

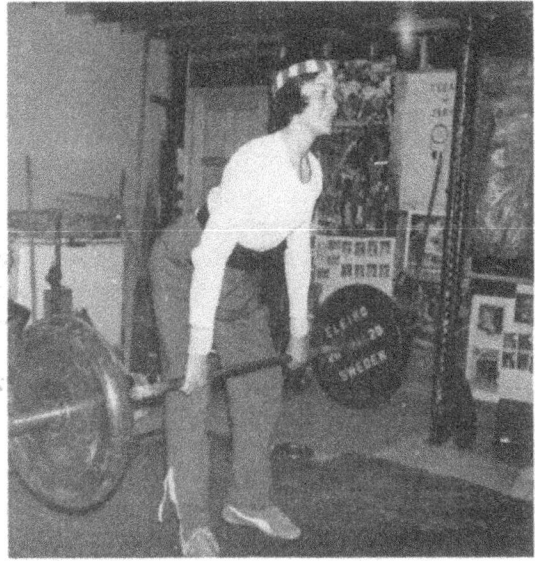

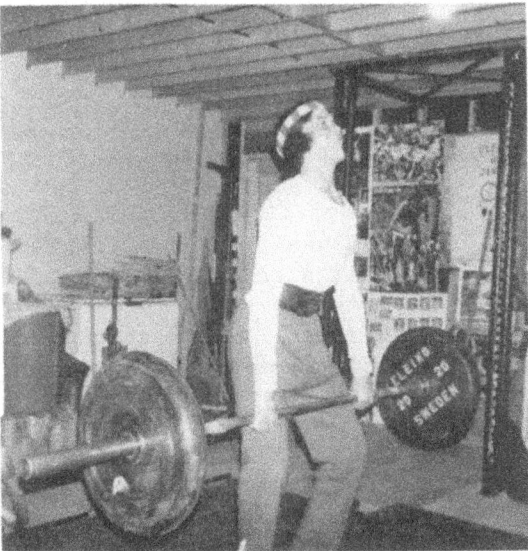

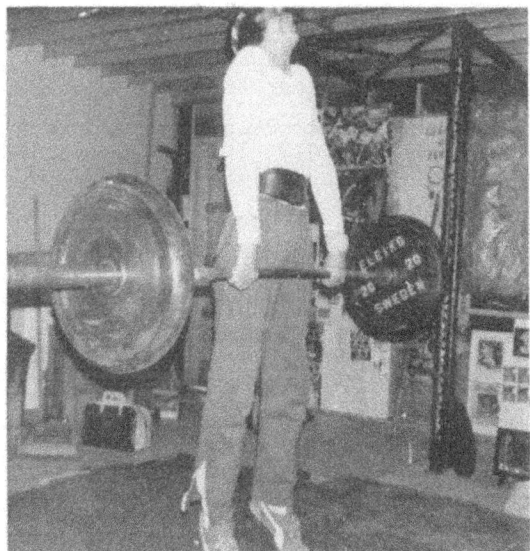

Exercise #6 - Olympic Dead Lift, Scoop and Shrug

Pulling - Bulgaria #4

The pulling technique known as the double knee bend, which we have been trying to explain and teach, was elaborated on by the different coaches at the European Coaches' Conference in Sofia, Bulgaria. I received insight as to how we might better describe and teach it in our country when I stayed on an extra day after the conference was over and had a four hour interview with the head coach of the Bulgarian team, Ivan Abadjeav.

It was discussed that Kolev, for example, seems to yank the bar off the floor. This is not exactly what is wanted. Rather, the lifter should make as fast a start as possible with the leverage at hand. The increasing of the speed should take place all along the pull as optimum leverage points are reached and succeeding speed is built on what went before. This is different from deliberately pulling slow off the floor. The lifter should make use of every leverage point. He should not yank the bar in an effort to get speed and he should not break good body positions. In other words, the lifter should go as fast as the leverage at hand will permit with good body position.

The fact that muscle loses contractile force rapidly when contracted fast does not have a negative influence on what has just been said. The rebending of the knees, or scooping, accomplishes three things: 1) A stretch-reflex action takes place, something like when a basketball player dips quickly to jump. This makes the quadriceps muscles contract harder than they could normally be called upon to do. 2) The rebending allows the muscles previously contracting to "rest" since they are no longer contracting to cause the upward movement, but are eccentrically controlling the hips and thighs down and forward. 3) It dramatically shifts the angle of pull so that even though the muscle has lost much of its contractile force since it has contracted rapidly, the angle of pull is so much better because of the scoop that it more than makes up for what the muscle has lost. (This is an important point. Whenever a choice must be made as to what is more important for power, angle of pull or strength of muscle, angle of pull outweighs the influence of strength of muscle.) These things combined with increased mementum of the bar make for a more powerfull overall pull.

In discussing the direction the bar should be pulled, it was pointed out that theoretically it is desirable for the bar to be pulled in a straight line so that the straight forces add up to a bigger resultant force than the total of forces going in different directions. However, this is not possible since the bar starts from over the metatarsals and must be brought in. A deviation of five centimeters or two inches is thought to be all right and will not cause swing. It might be argued that if the bar were placed right next to the ankles then it could be pulled straight up. But if this were done, the bodyweight would be centered back on the heels instead of the middle front of the foot. With the bodyweight thus centered further back, the natural rotation of the back, even if done perfectly, would cause the bodyweight to go even further back behind the heels; then the lifter would jump back and probably swing the bar. So the bar has got to be started from the metatarsal part of the foot and "pulled in". This pulling in should be, as mentioned, five centimeters or two inches. It is more dramatic in the Bulgarian manner of pulling than in the Russian manner. In the Bulgarian style it is almost hooked in or cradled in, whereas in the Russian style, it is pulled in on a gradual plane. In either case, it should not be beyond the five centimeters or two inches, or else a swing will develop. In some of the Bulgarian lifters, this unwanted swing has developed and is trying to be worked out. To help correct this, a machine is now being used with the Bulgarian Senior National Team which measures the distance the bar is pulled in. The machine also measures the direction of the bar and the height it reaches. It has worked well with the junior teams and it is hoped it will now help the senior team.

In starting off the floor, when anatomically feasible (usually with a lifter of long upper thigh), the lifter should have his hips higher than parallel to the floor. This is for three reasons: 1) With the hips higher, the weight of the bar is more apt to be directed up instead of back. 2) With the hips higher, the thighs are in better leverage position to exert maximum force (it is easier to do a squat than a half squat), and since the legs are one of the prime movers in coming off the floor, they should be in the best leverage or position. 3) With the hips higher, the lever arm (where the bar would intersect with the spine) will be decreased, since the back will be lower.

In getting the hips higher than parallel, the lifter should maintain shoulder width stance with the feet slightly pointed out. A wider stance than this makes the hips drop. Also, a wide stance means that the bar is not pulled as high as with a shoulder width or narrower stance since the lifter stands lower with a wider stance. Having the feet slightly pointed out gets more of the legs into the pull.

Every effort should be made to not have the knees spread apart when the pull is done because the knees going out means that the hips drop. This causes backward movement of the bar, allows the back to come upright too soon, and thus increases the lever arm (previously explained).

In discussion about the wrists, it was pointed out that in the snatch and the clean, the less swing at the top, the better; for this reason, it is desirable to keep the wrists flexed. This throws the elbows forward and out to the sides. Besides facilitating an upright rowing motion instead of a back rowing motion, this flexion of the wrists and resulting throwing of the elbows forward and out makes the traps stretch more, thus having a stronger effect on the bar. Also, the traps react more strongly since a muscle on stretch contracts stronger than when it is not on stretch. Finally, having the elbows thrown forward and out makes the traps pull the weight up and the scapula raise full distance up the ribs. If the elbows were back, then the traps would not be able to lift up the scapula efficiently and the rhomboids would then take the dominant role and pull the scapula back, thus cutting down on the pull. For the same reason, the head should not be thrown back at the top. As the back comes into play, the head is tossed back but then is tucked in at the top of the pull. To have it still going back at the top means not only will the scapula not go up as far as possible, but also a final rotation backward would be apt to result.

Jerk Techniques and Exercises

In recent years much attention has been focused on the jerk because of its de-
creasing success following the dropping of the press from competition. The important basics of a successful jerk have been scrutinized with some previous concepts
being dropped, some being sustained and some being added to. Certainly more concepts will evolve as it has been only a few years that such scrutiny has taken
place. In this article will be presented some concepts both new and old that have
thus far come out as being on solid ground.

The main power for the jerk comes from the hips and thighs. Shoulder strength
is needed for support for stability to insure constant contact of the shoulders
with the bar as it rests on the shoulders throughout the dip and drive. Shoulder
strength is also needed from hair line level to the full extension in order to push
the body rapidly under the bar and to lock properly underneath the weight.

When the bar is on the shoulders the elbows should be directed at an angle to
the side and pointing slightly below horizontal. This position has proven to be
the strongest from practical experience and also from cable tension tests on the
supporting muscles of the shoulder and upper arm.

The head and eyes are slightly tilted up, and in some cases the head is tucked
back. A compact feeling should be felt all across the shoulder and chest area. To
ensure this, the chest is thought of as being high. It may or may not appear this
way depending on the development of the chest of the lifter. The adductors and ab-
ductors of the upper arm are contracted to stabilize the upper arm when the bar is
at the shoulders, during the dip and the drive.

The center of gravity of the body should pass from the shoulders down through
the ankle bone if the lifter is standing upright. If the rear end is slightly
tilted back then the center of gravity is slightly forward. Assuming that the
lifter is standing upright, he dips four to six inches straight down with the hips
level. If the lifter dips with his hips slightly to the back, then the four to six
inch dip will be with hips slightly tilted back with the pelvis tilted to the front.
There is also the lifter who dips the four to six inches with his hips slightly to
the back and then rotates them till they are level on the drive up. This last type
of lifter is using a rotary drive.

Since I have alluded to three different types of accepted dips, I would like
to discuss them a little. The lifter who dips straight down with his hips right
underneath him will have the center of gravity go well towards the front when he
dips. The weight will be felt on the middle of the front thigh. With this type of
dip the extension upward is straight and powerful and well-positioned.

The lifter who dips with rear end slightly tilted back (pelvis tipping forward
of horizontal) has to make sure his drive does not go forward. The tilt of the pelvis should remain stable and not increase. A lifter who dips this way sometimes
has a tight sacro-iliac joint, and to ask him to push his rear end in (pelvis horizontal) usually result in pain in this joint. With his rear end slightly tilted
back, as he dips the weight is felt more in the hips and upper front of the thighs.
The center of gravity when he dips will not go as far forward as it does for the
previous lifter described. A lifter who lifts this way has been very successful in
the past because he drives the weight so powerfully with the hips slightly back. He
has to watch that he does not drive the weight forward, as mentioned before. One

thing he can do is to keep his lower back as flexible as possible. Another thing he can do is to really move the front foot well forward in the split. (I will say more on this later.)

When discussing the previous lifter, I am not talking about the lifter whose rear end is way back and goes even farther back when he dips so that he constantly throws the weight out front. I am talking about the lifter whose natural tilt of the pelvis is such that the rear end is only slightly tilted back and represents no major problem as long as other things are watched and adhered to.

The final type of dip I mentioned is the one which imparts a rotary drive up. This is a very unique type of drive, and more will have to be learned about rotary motion of the human body in order to say whether or not it is a superior technique. However, there are some advantages which are readily apparent. When this lifter dips, his rear end is slightly tilted back. As the drive starts, the rear is still tilted back. This results in a much stronger drive up than if the hips were level to begin with. This has been proven on force plate machines and can be seen on the read-out dial on the slow speed of an Isokinetic Power Rack. After a short moment the hips are brought in and forward so that they are underneath the upper body. With this style there exists the possibility that the lifter gets the best of both worlds. He gets a stronger drive and he drives the weight straight up. Whether there is any loss of power in the rotary action itself is a subject for further study. In any case, some lifters in our country are using this rotary action and some of the international stars are also using it.

The lifter using this style gets another advantage, namely, by pushing the hips in a rotary type style the hips have momentum travelling forward. This allows the lifter's upper body to lean back, which in turn allows for facilitation in reaching out with the front foot, and it also allows for easy clearance of the head by the bar.

An aspect of the dip applicable to all three methods should be mentioned. Sometimes in the dip an instability is felt. A conscious pinching or adduction of the glutes (rear) will help overcome this feeling. An instability can also be felt not only during the dip but also while supporting the weight before the dip and while supporting the weight when the bar is overhead if there is no stability around the waist area. This means that strong muscles are needed in this area. Usually the lower back is strong enough, but where strength may be lacking is in the abdominal muscles and oblique muscles.

Something else applicable to all methods of dipping is flexibility in the ankles. No matter what method is used, the bodyweight has got to shift forward, and this will be more difficult with a lack of flexibility in the ankles. If this is lacking, then the lifter has a tendency to push from the back center of the foot, and this results in a strong possibility of driving the weight forward. Also, to reach a four to six inch dip with the hips underneath or the hips slightly in back (but remaining stable throughout the dip), a lifter has to have flexible ankles. All this is because the foreleg has got to go well forward in the dip. It can if there is good flexibility in the ankles, and it will not if there is not. If ankle flexibility is lacking, then the body usually inclines forward in the dip with the rear shooting out back; the resultant drive will throw the bar in front or the dip will not be low enough to get proper leverage for maximum drive. In trying to keep upright or maintain stable hip position when dipping, the body cannot dip low enough with inflexible ankles.

The positioning of the feet when the bar is at the shoulders is a subject of discussion. While there are some lifters who place their toes straight ahead, many

27

have their feet pointing slightly out. This results in greater force being used by the total quadriceps. This has been shown on force plate machines and in connection with electromyographs.

It is very important to dip four to six inches. Any more or less results in less leverage for maximum thrust of the hips and legs. Most lifters are able to dip the four to six inches by using a stance about equal in width to the shoulders. Some lifters find this dip difficult; they usually go too low or are inconsistent in their depth of dip. In this case a narrow stance will keep the lifter from going lower. This is usually accompanied by the toes pointing toward the front which further prevents going lower. Wide stances have been experimented with but without too much success to date.

The speed of the dip should be controlled. Neither an extra slow or an extra fast dip is wanted. The thinking is that the lifter will usually find out his own best speed. The bar used makes a difference, especially when heavy weights are used. With a less springy bar, the lifter can dip faster, and with a more springy bar the lifter should dip slower. Also, with a less springy bar the lifter should dip farther, and with a more springy bar he should dip less.

When the four to six inch drop is reached, with the hips level or slightly back, a violent but controlled upward thrust takes place by the extension of the hips and legs. As stated before, an extension straight upward is wanted, not out in front. If the bar goes out in front, then it is usually because the hips have gone farther back in the dip or in the drive upward; thus in the drive up the body inclines forward and is not vertical. In the rotary drive the same effect is wanted, an extension upward, not out in front. Another cause of a forward drive is the center of gravity of the body staying back. Even with the hips underneath or at a slight tilt or in the rotary action, a lifter can "get trapped on his heels". If the body inclines forward but the hips do not go further back and the shoulder area is stable and does not change position, then it is possible that the lifter is driving off his heels instead of the whole foot, so the weight goes out front. Also, if he is driving off of his heels, he will not be able to extend on his toes as easily, if at all.

As the drive continues it is a must that the lifter extends all the way up on his toes. We hear of cutting the pull short. Well, many lifters cut the drive of the jerk short. This is usually because they split before they fully extend on their toes.

After the lifter has extended on his toes and as he is splitting, he leans back slightly. This lean back: 1) helps the front foot move well ahead because it takes most of the restriction away from getting the front foot out as far as desired (if the lifter were leaning forward instead, the front foot would have restrictions placed on it and it would be harder to get it out far enough), 2) helps drive the hips under the weight, and 3) helps the bar clear the head.

World records have been jerked without a lean back as just described, but I subscribe to the lean back because of its many advantages. However, a lifter who has a big forward tilt of the pelvis so that the rear end sticks out quite a bit may have trouble doing this because the sacroiliac joint is formed so that this tilt forward takes place. For such a lifter to lean back may not be possible because of pain since the joint when formed this way does not want to go in that direction and/or because there is not sufficient flexibility to permit this. I advise staying as loose as possible in the sacroiliac joint in order to possibly use this lean back style or at the very least to prevent injury in that joint since many stresses are put on it which seem to accentuate this tilt forward, and nothing much is done to lessen the stresses. Flexibility work will lessen the stresses.

The bar being driven off of the shoulders should go to the hairline level; this is the height needed to successfully push oneself underneath a jerk. Any higher is usually wasted height and motion unless a lifter is not flexible and/or is slow and needs the extra height. As this height is being reached, the elbows come out a little more to the side. This elbow position while the bar is at the hairline level should be the same as when the bar was at that level during the press (when that lift was being contested). This is a very strong angle for the lifter to push himself underneath the weight, and pushing himself under the weight with the bar in such a position is what the lifter wants to do. He cannot drive the weight farther up because he has extended on his toes. He must push himself underneath the weight with speed and force so that he can get a good position for a solid support of the weight overhead.

In pushing himself under the bar, the lifter should reach up and out with his arms. This locks the arm better at the elbow and where the upper arm fits into the scapula. It also fixes the scapula better on the ribs. In doing this the elbows will turn to the outside. Merely to push up so that the elbows are straightened is not enough; many a heavy jerk has come down because there was not supportive leverage of the weight. The lifter should be thinking of pushing himself down, and as the elbows reach a straightened position, he should reach up and turn the elbows to the outside, at the same time thinking of stretching the bar out.

The chest, which is held high when the bar is at the shoulders and during the dip and the drive, should be kept high and should move forward. Lifters and coaches talk about "forcing the chest through" on the jerk. This is really a must if the weight overhead is going to be adequately supported. If the chest is not "forced through", then the weight is not only less stable overhead, but also it is not overhead where it should be (a little behind the head is permissable); instead it is out in front.

The split fore and aft should be close to the ground. Almost a shuffle is wanted, but without friction from the floor. A minimal distance between the lifter's feet and the floor is wanted during this "shuffle". Any more is a waste of time in the air and loss of time in positioning underneath the bar.

The split should be long. In past years it was advocated that the front foot travel one measure for every two measures of the back foot. Now the thinking is that the front foot should travel one and a half measures for every two measures of the back foot. For the lifter with a big forward tilt of the pelvis this will seem like an especially long distance, and getting the front foot out will be harder. With the pelvis tilted forward, the front foot comes down quicker, something like a long jumper who is tilted forward in the air; his feet come down quicker.

With this further reach by the front foot, a 90° angle or more between the upper leg and lower leg is formed and is wanted. This is because more fore and aft mobility can take place with a heavy weight and a better leverage angle is obtained than if an acute angle (less than 90°) were formed. With an acute angle it is difficult to maneuver fore and aft, and recovery with heavy weights is harder because of poorer leverage. Also, with a 90° angle or more, a wider base of support is gained, which means more stability.

The back knee can be slightly bent because it will not buckle with this elongated stance. The heel can be off the floor. With the back knee bent and the heel off the floor, the lifter can more easily adjust his body weight than if the back knee were straight and the heel on the floor. Also, with the back knee bent and

29

the heel off the floor, the lifter can adjust for the uneven timing of the placement of the feet fore and aft in the split. The front and back feet should be in
their place at the same time. If the back knee were straight and the heel on the
floor, the late placement of the front foot would cause such a jar and the supporting structure of the legs would be so rigid that the jerk would stand a good chance
of coming down.

It should be mentioned that although the placement of the feet in the split
should be at the same time, uneven placement sometimes occurs. If the back foot is
in its place first, with the back knee bent and the heel off the floor, the lifter
can sink and cushion the impact of the later placement of the front foot. The back
foot placing first is easier to adjust to because there is not so much strain with
a long split. A sinking motion of the front foot is harder to do because there is
more concentration of force felt on that leg than on the back leg, and the lifter
usually resists this sinking of the front foot because he feels such a loss of leverage. This is a very uneasy feeling with a heavy weight overhead. However, with
a 90° angle or an obtuse angle between the upper leg and lower leg of the front
foot, this sinking feeling produces less loss of leverage than if an acute angle
were formed. By leaning back as he splits the lifter ensures that if any uneven
placement is going to take place, it will be the back foot that is placed first in
the split position, not the front.

The toes of the front foot are turned in slightly to prevent slipping, and the
back toes can be turned slightly out for the same reason. Some lifters believe in
turning the back toes slightly in, but this throws the weight on the outside of the
foot which is shorter and offers less support. By turning the toes slightly out,
support is thrown on the longer inside of the foot which means more support. Slippage does take place too often because of uneven support. The positioning of the
feet as just described will help prevent some slippage. If the support is too uneven then very little can be done to prevent slipping.

With heavy weights overhead one must be very careful during recovery. It is
known that many world records are recovered with one step back and one step forward
and with the feet coming high off the floor. It can be done, but every once in a
while a heavy jerk is lost while taking such steps. It may be that the jerk is positioned wrong or it is so heavy and the lifter so low that with that much distance
to be covered by only one step back and one step forward, too much base of support
is lost for that heavy a weight in that position, and the jerk comes down. Or it
may be that by picking the front foot up high off the ground and also the back foot,
too much time is spent in the air with no base of support, so again the jerk comes
down. The lifter should take two steps back with the front foot, actually shuffling
or sliding back, and then he takes one step forward with the back foot, again with
the foot close to the ground.

In any case it is usually incorrect to recover with the back foot first. Too
many jerks are thrown forward from their base of support and dropped. However, an
exception to this is the lifter with a pronounced tilt of the pelvis; he might have
to recover back to front. This is because there is so much weight concentrated on
the front foot that it is impossible to pick up. This forward tilt is because of
the structural formation of the sacroiliac joint. This type of lifter should be
careful about several things. One is that he must be quick. Pushing from back to
front means that even more weight is going to be forward, and until a solid base of
support is gained there is going to be a lot of instability with the weight wanting
to come down in front. If the lifter is not quick, then he will not be able to gain
stability in time. Another thing is that he must keep pushing up and out; the lifter will need this bone on bone leverage more than ever since the stability is uncer-
tain. Finally, he must keep coming up. That means that the body should be rising

30

up when coming forward, not sinking. If the lifter recovers forward and sinks, he
will be driven down; he must rise.

There is a style taught by the American coach, Joe Mills, in which the lifter
is taught to recover back to front. Joe tells me that he only teaches it when the
conventional style does not work and if the lifter is quick. An analysis of this
style brings out certain merits. The lifter drives the weight up and then runs under it, pushing off the back foot, reaching up as much as possible. What this means
is that before the weight has slowed down, the lifter is exerting force up from his
run up to the bar which is still going up. The lifter has to be quick because if
he is not, then when he runs up and under the bar and reaches up, he is going to be
pushed down by the weight which has started its descent. But if the lifter is
quick enough, he will catch the bar as it is still going up, and his going up will
add to the upward motion of the bar.

All Pictures but Starred Ones by Klemens

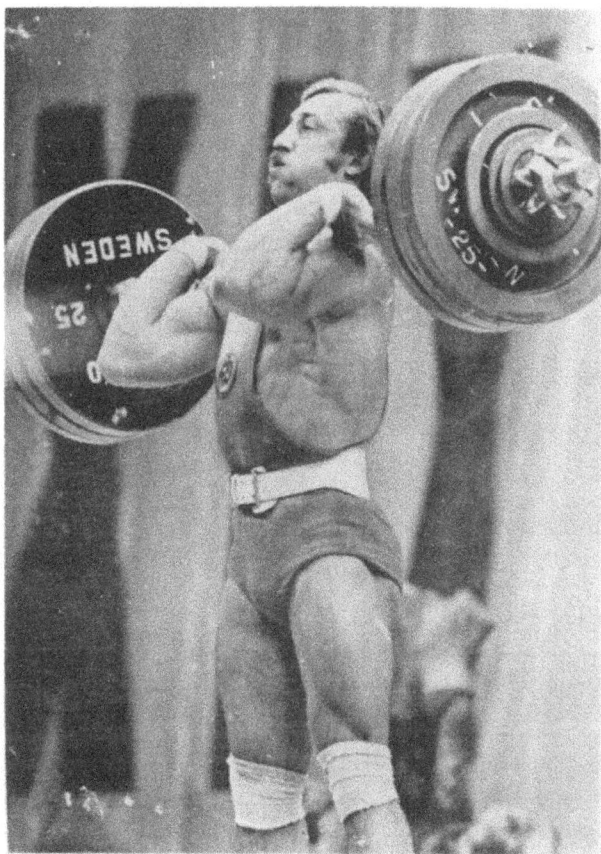

* #1 Elbows slightly down and slightly out
    to side; head slightly up; solid con-
    tact of bar with shoulders; rear end
    slightly tilted back.

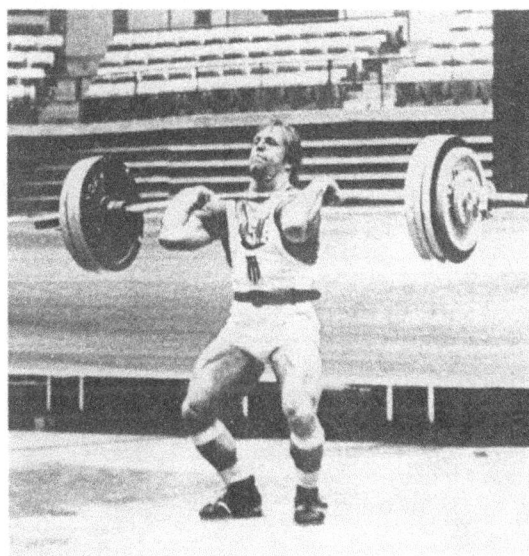

#2 This lifter has rear end tucked
   in during 4-6" dip; weight felt
   on mid-front of thighs; feet
   shoulder distance apart, slightly
   turned out; elbows slightly down
   and slightly out to side; head
   slightly up.

31

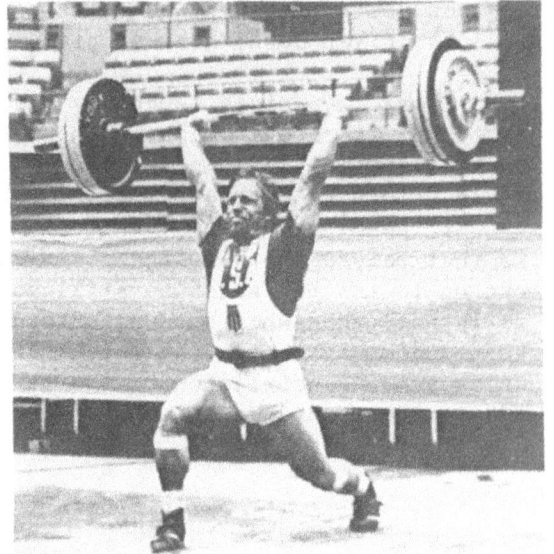

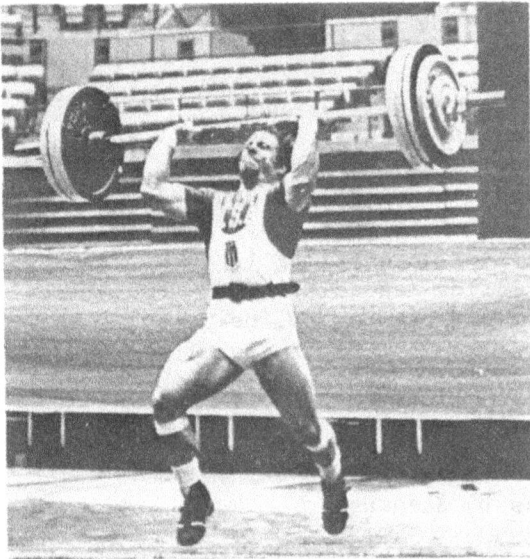

#3 Bar driven to hairline level; lifter
leaning back, pushing himself under
bar; elbows slightly out to side;
feet too high off floor.

#4 Lifter pushing up and out on bar;
elbows to side; front foot 90° angle
or more and turned slightly in; back
toes turned slightly out for support
from long side of foot; back heel
off floor; back knee bent.

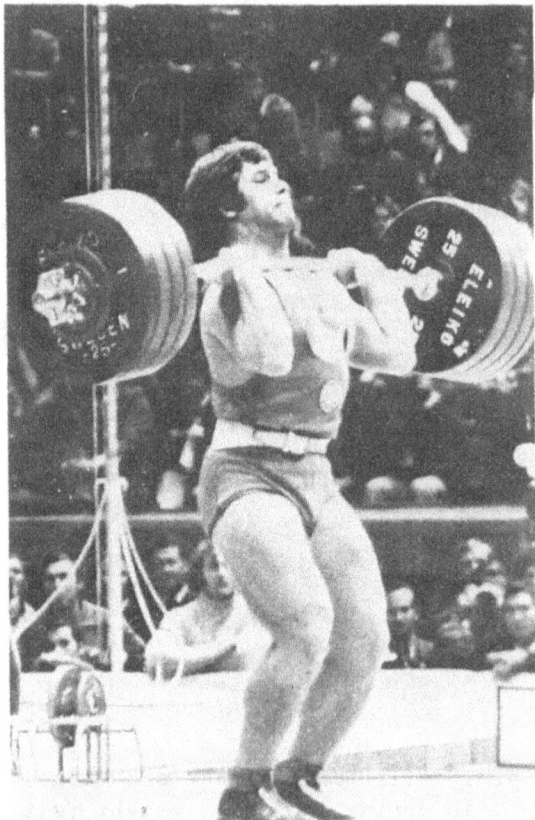

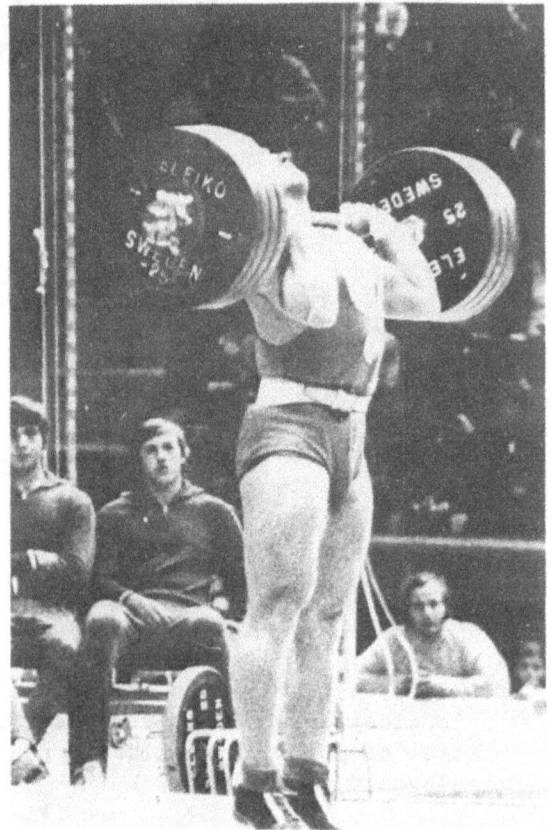

#5 Lifter dipping with rear slightly
out (okay if not increased); weight
felt on hips and top part of thighs;
lifter will time bend of bar to aid
his drive.

#6 Good extension on balls of feet; direc-
tion of extension straight up; bar is
whipping up.

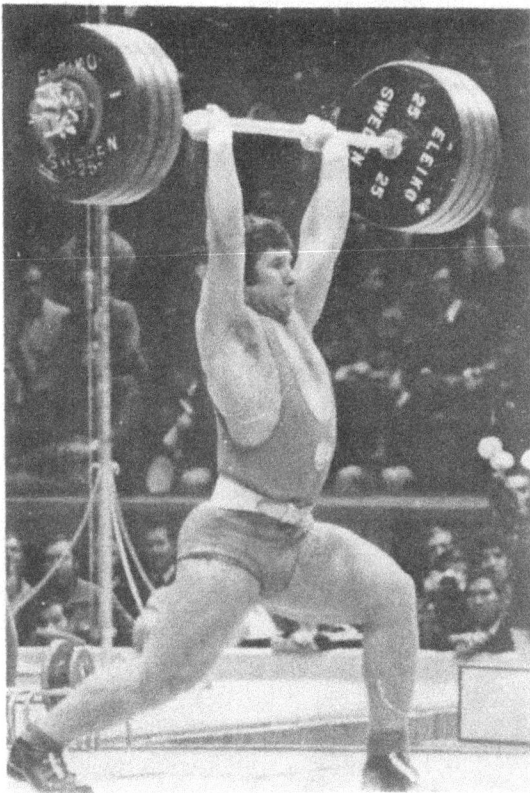

#7 Good split with front leg 90° angle or
more; chest up; lifter has not reached
up and out with arms; a lot of muscles
holding bar instead of bone support.

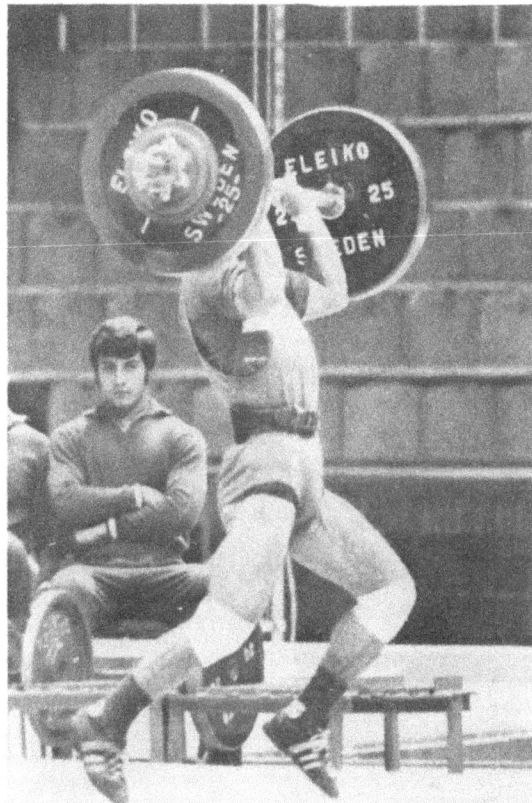

#8 Note strong elbow position to side
which allows strong push under bar;
lifter leaning back; feet going front
and back close to floor, not in air.

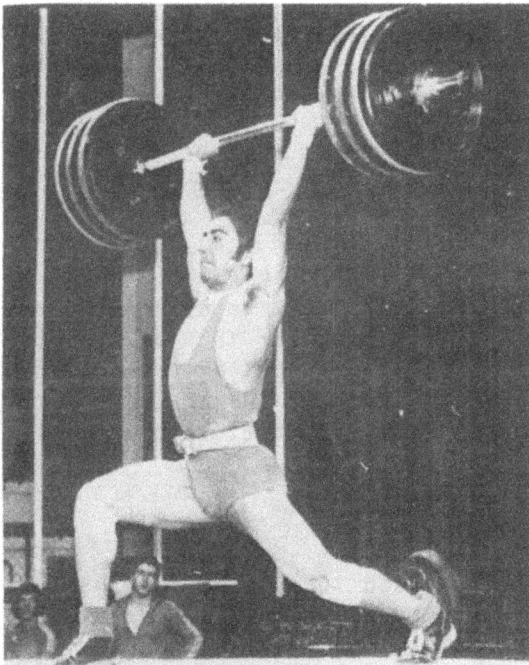

* #9 Lifter has reached up and out; good
bone support; front foot 90° angle or
more; stance elongated; chest up and
through; back knee safely bent and heel
safely off floor.

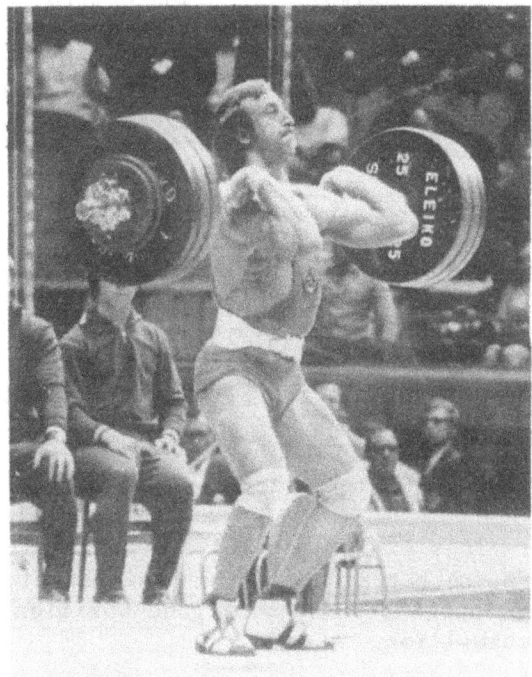

#10 Rotary Drive: Dip is with hips
slightly back.

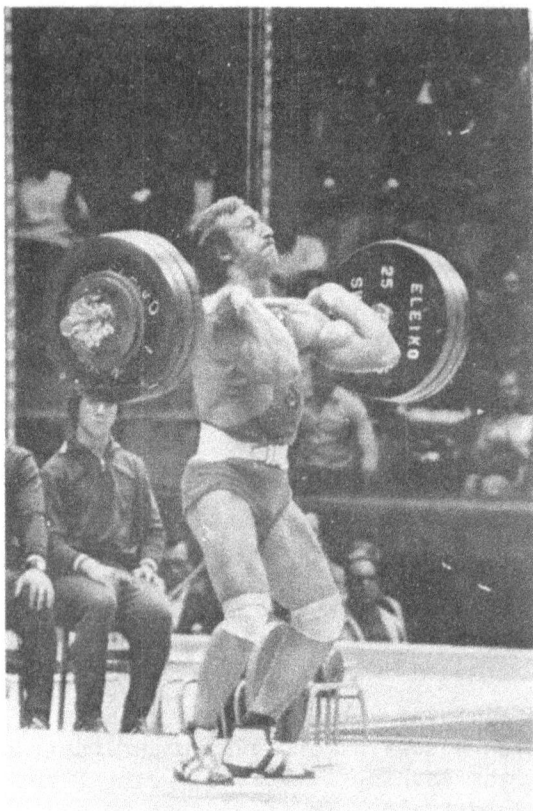

#11 Rotary Drive: Hips come forward; note
    distance between hips and loader's
    arm here and in #10; bodyweight goes
    forward; weight felt shifts to lower-
    front thigh from up higher.

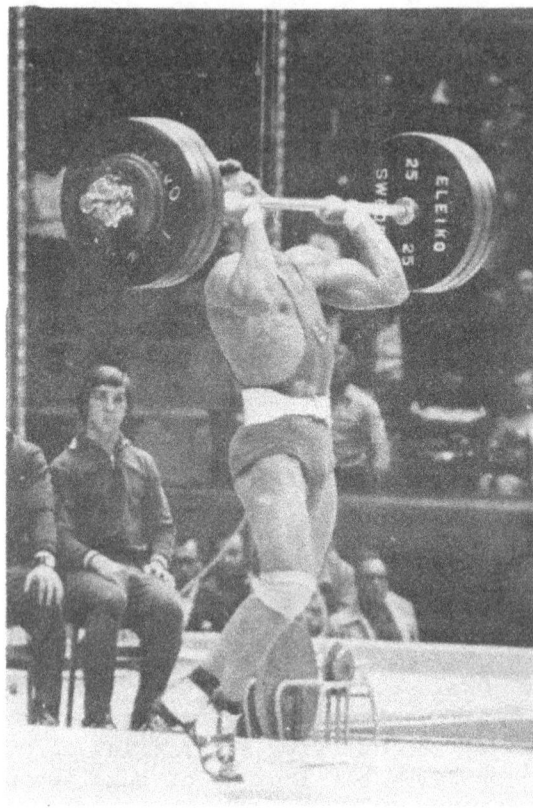

#12 Rotary Drive: Hips go farther for-
    ward (using same focal point) and
    up; upper body leans back.

Jerk Exercises

While more can be said concerning jerk style, for this short paper I would now like to explain a few of the better exercises that can be used for the jerk. Four will be demonstrated by pictures at the end. Reps of the different exercises, intensities and loads will be discussed in some of the articles in the Training Methods section. Correct jerk style should be used in all full or partial motions of the exercises.

On Toes, Split and Recover

This exercise teaches awareness of pushing on extended toes, good body position when the bar is at its highest height, the feeling of pushing oneself under a weight, good splitting methods, good position when under the bar, and strength in the recovery position.

With the bar resting on pins between supports at hairline level, the lifter is positioned on his toes as he would be after the drive which carries the bar to hairline level. With the lifter under the bar, he then recovers. During the whole exercise the lifter should have a coach or fellow lifter check for good form (or as a last resort, he himself can do it) as explained earlier.

Push Up and Out

This exercise develops strength in the shoulders as needed in the part of the jerk where the lifter pushes himself under a weight. With the bar resting on the pins between the supports at hairline height or higher, the lifter pushes the bar up. As the bar gets to the extended position, the lifter continues to push up and turns his elbows out. Merely pushing the bar to the extended position is not enough. The lifter must push up farther and turn his elbows out.

Jerk Drive

This exercise develops power for the jerk and also develops the correct bottom dip position and final drive position where the lifter is extended upward on his toes. With the bar resting on the pins between the supports at a height about one inch below the regular dip of the lifter (this is to take into account the sinking in of the bar to the flesh), the lifter positions himself under the weight exactly as he would be at the bottom of the dip for the jerk. He then drives the weight off the pins so that the bar reaches hairline level. The lifter should extend on his toes. He then guides the bar down to the pins; he does not let it drop onto his shoulders. Because of the crashing of the bar on the pins, an old bar should be used.

Jerk Balance

This exercise is designed especially for the lifter who does not step forward with his front foot. A semi-split position is taken. A dip from this position is made and the weight is driven to hairline level, and then the lifter moves his front foot forward. The back foot does not move.

Jerk Push or Push Jerk

This exercise teaches the lifter to drive hard, extend all the way, pushing up and out with the shoulders and arms. It has been called many things, and even its present name is misleading since there should be no press. It should be driven to arms' length. With the bar on the chest in a normal jerk position, the lifter drives the weight up high enough so that he pushes himself under the bar with no split.

There are two ideas on foot movement during this. One is to have the feet remain stationary after going on his toes. The other is to have the feet skip to the side. With the feet skipping to the side, more weight can be handled. If the lifter extends all the way up, this might be better since more weight can be handled. If the lifter seems to be sneaking under the weight and not driving it up, then he should not have the feet going to the side.

Jerk, Eyes Closed

This is done exactly like a normal jerk taken off the rack except that the eyes are closed. It is known that a person deprived of one of his senses develops the others more fully. Many times the jerk coordination pattern is developed by doing this exercise when all else fails.

Special Waist Exercises for the Jerk

Back Oblique Raise

The lifter lies face down slightly on his side at a 45° angle, with his rear end near the end of the bench and his feet well supported. He lets his body go all the way down, then raises up until his body is above parallel; he does 10-15 reps. Then he turns on the other side and does the same for 10-15 reps. He holds his hands across his chest. If more weight is needed, then he holds this weight at his chest.

Front Oblique Raise

This is done the same as the back oblique raise except the lifter lies face up.

Twisting Leg Raise

The lifter assumes a position as if he were going to do normal leg raises. He raises his knees and twists them to one side. Then he extends his legs as his body lands on that side. Now he repeats the action, twisting all the way over to the other side. This is one repetition since both sides have been acted on. He does 14-20 reps. Resistance is added by increasing the angle of incline or by putting weights on the feet.

Bent-Knee Sit-Ups

The lifter does sit-ups with the knees well bent so that less than a 90° angle is formed between the upper and lower legs. The arms are across his chest. If weight is needed it is put on the chest. Increased resistance can also be gotten by increasing the angle of the incline. The lifter should not do the sit-ups with a flat back; he should curl up, until his head touches his knee. He does 15-20 reps.

Knee-Ups

Sitting on the edge of a bench, the lifter grasps the bench leaning slightly forward, maintaining this lean as he brings his knees to his chest. He does 15-20 reps. Weight can be added to the feet for increased resistance.

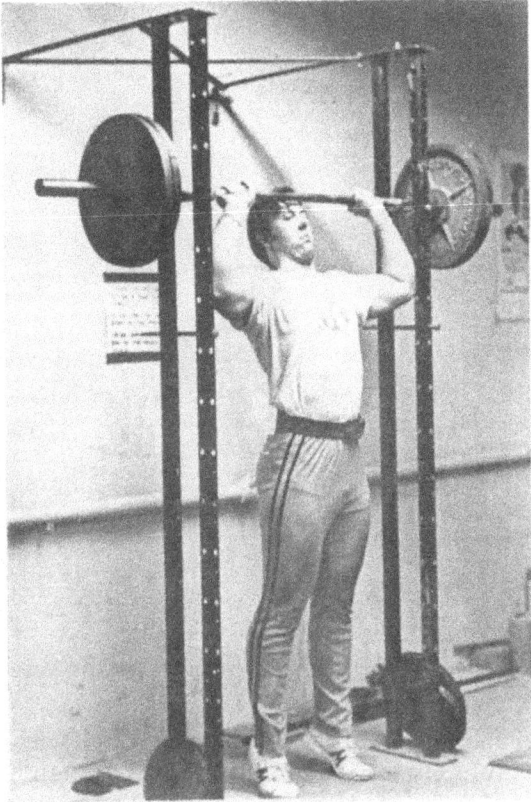

#1 <u>On Toes, Split & Recover</u> - Lifter is positioned as he would be after the drive which takes the bar to hairline level. Elbows are a little too much to the side.

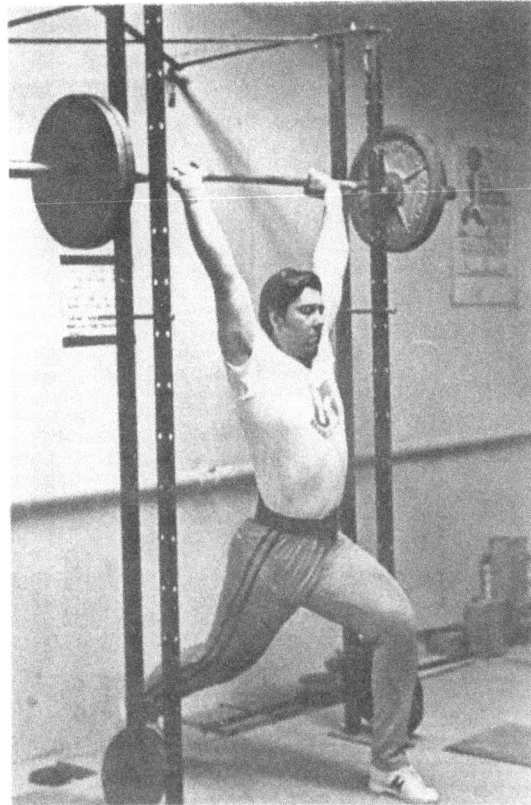

#2 <u>On Toes, Split & Recover</u> - Lifter has pushed himself underneath the weight, pushing up and out on the bar. From this position he will recover to a standing position.

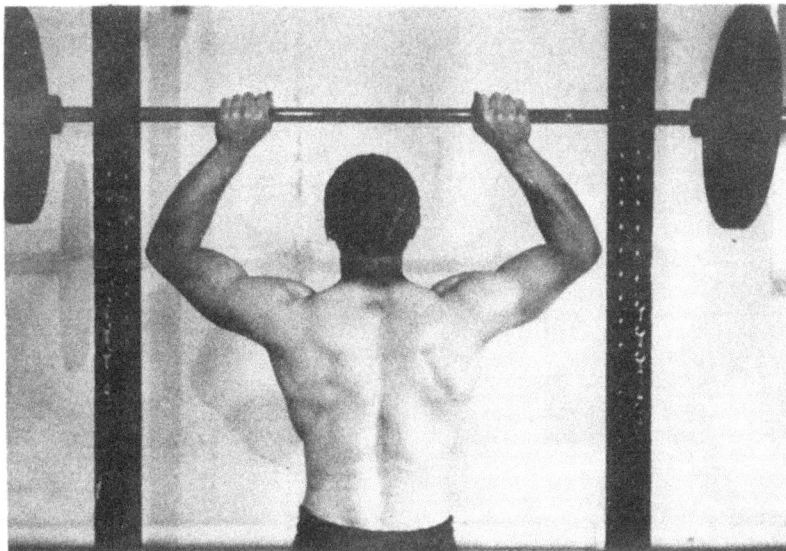

#3 <u>Push Up & Out</u> - From height of hairline or above, lifter positions himself under the bar in vertical position, ready to push up on bar.

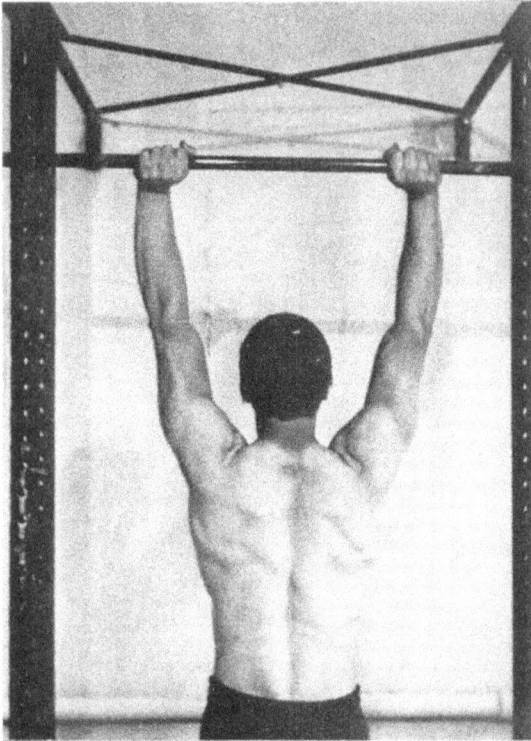

#4 Push Up & Out - Remaining vertical, lifter pushed up on bar. Note elbows, shoulders and traps and compare them with the next picture.

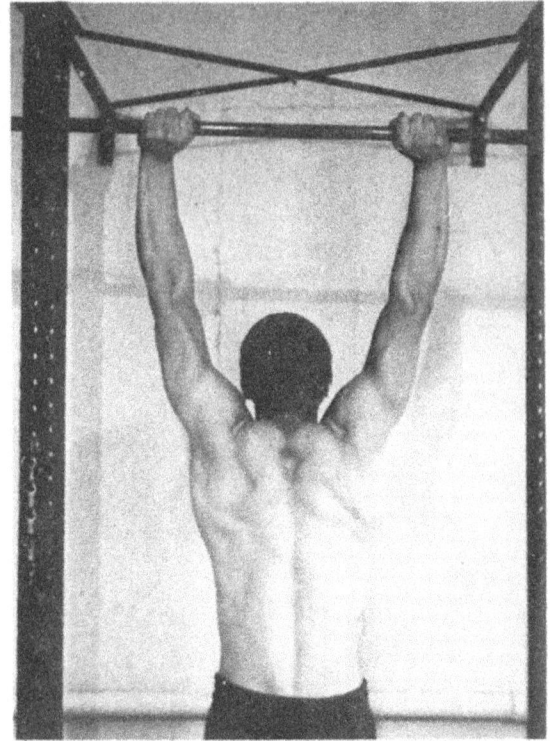

#5 Push Up & Out - From previous position lifter has continued to push up and also <u>out</u> on bar. Note elbows have moved not only out but a little back, and traps and shoulders are higher. This, not photo #4 position, is the strongest position to support a weight overhead.

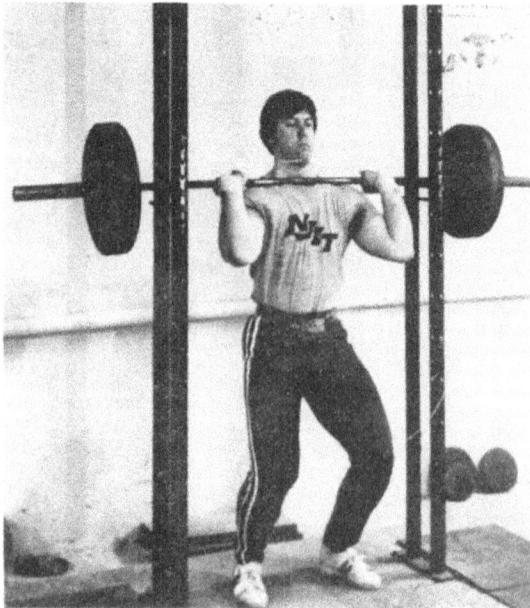

#6 Jerk Drive - With bar resting on rack, lifter assumes position he would be in at bottom of the dip for the jerk.

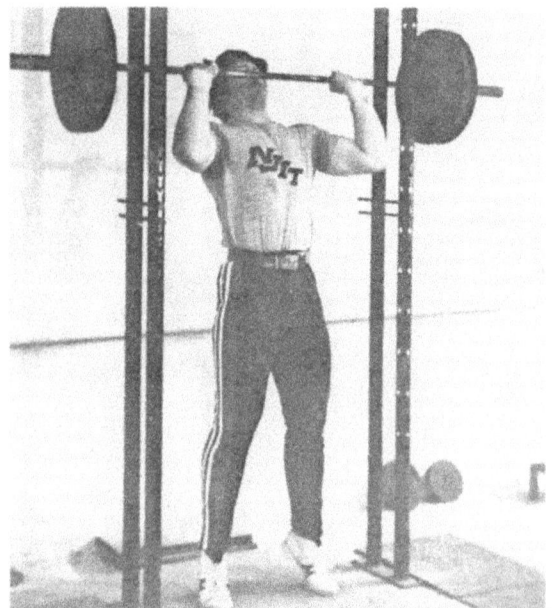

#7 Jerk Drive - Lifter has driven bar so it will go to hairline level. He is up on his toes.

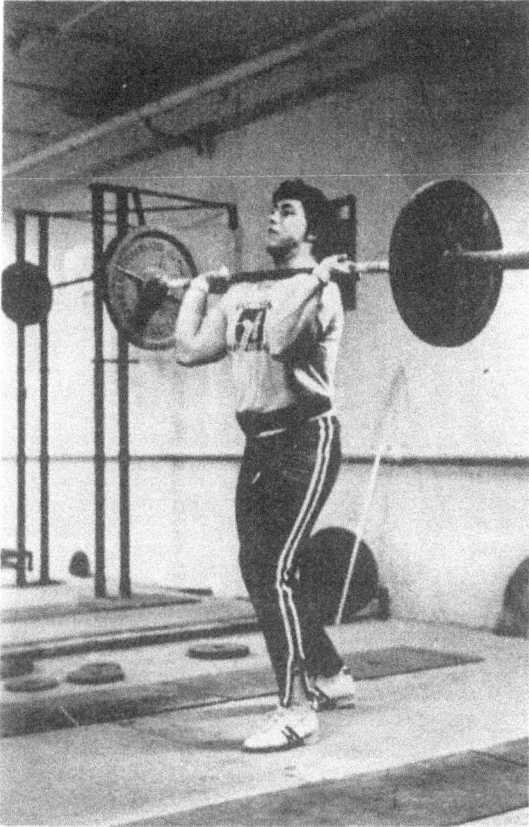

#8 <u>Jerk Balance</u> - Lifter dips for the jerk from semi-split position.

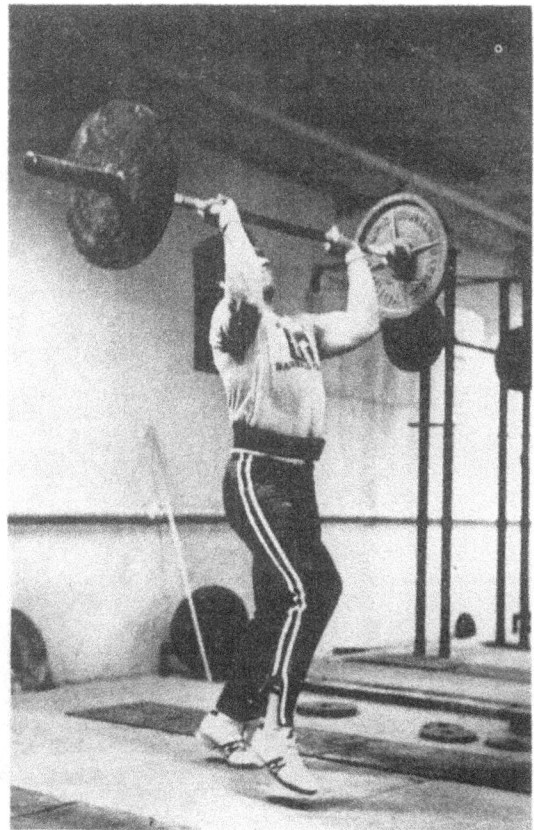

#9 <u>Jerk Balance</u> - With bar driven to hairline level, leaning back the lifter steps forward with only the front foot; back foot remains on floor. Front foot should just clear floor; it is too high here.

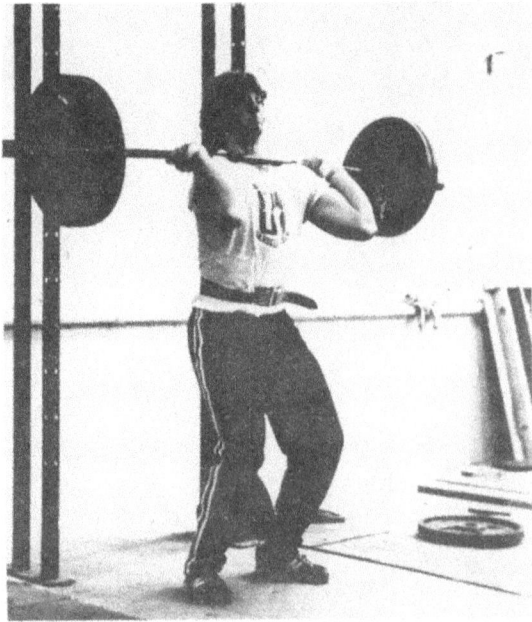

#10 <u>Push Jerk</u> - Lifter dips to drive weight up.

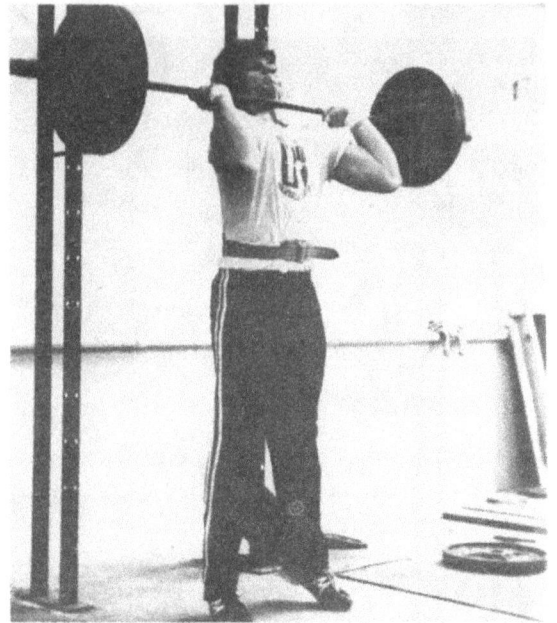

#11 <u>Push Jerk</u> - Lifter drives off his toes straight up.

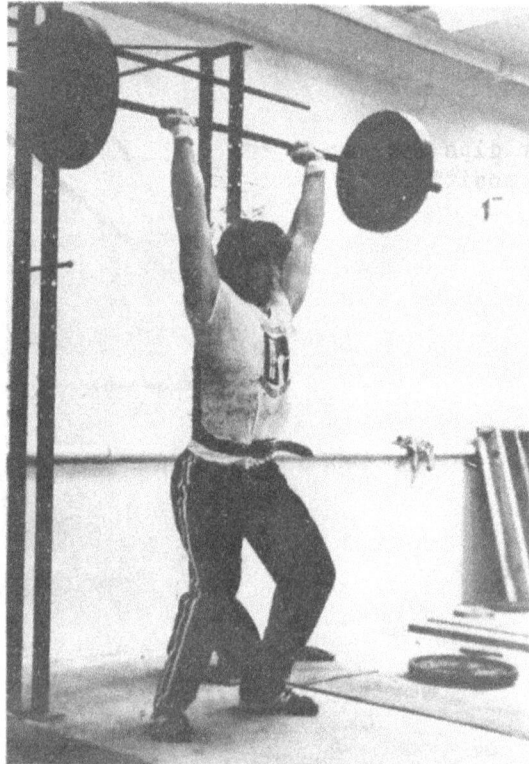

#12 <u>Push Jerk</u> - Lifter pushes himself under the weight, pushing up and out with the arms and shoulders.

Film Analysis

On the following pages are the analysis I did of two rolls of film, 250 feet each, which I shot when I was at the World Championships in Moscow. They are included in these writings because they point out some of the things that can be watched for when you are helping an athlete, and also they show how a film can be documented for use. These are general outlines of the two films. Any such film can be used in the same manner as a teaching tool.

1975 Moscow World Championships: Film #1

Opening Ceremony - girls go to stage with bread, and all IWF officers "break bread", symbolizing international goodwill through sports

114 lb. class competition - not worth describing; taken from too far away

little film taken of actual competition; most taken of training and the warm-up room

James (USA) - training; hips higher than parallel, shoulders in front of bar at knee (although could be more), good re-dip and excellent extension up

Grippaldi (USA) - training with high pulls; does not get shoulders over bar well at knees so when re-dips bar winds up in front of shoulders (shoulders in back of bar), therefore too much back and not enough leg and hip

old shot of Ivenchencov at 1970 Worlds in Columbus spliced in; short footage but put in to show tremendous extension he gets with shoulders; shoulders really do not go as much in front of bar as desirable when bar at knees, but he gets an upward extension because of tremendous coordination of getting bodyweight from back foot to front again, this being caused by really throwing knees and hips forward and up

Wentzel (E.Ger.) - training (in red shirt); starts a little soon when bar comes past knees so swings a little; on his misses they go out front when he really rushes pull; tries to force chest forward in jerk; steps out nice

Bonk (E.Ger) - training; misses snatch, rushes down on drop under; this usually does not happen as witnessed in other films; he usually shuffles under but in this case wasted time by jumping under; lot of other things right which are described better in other film

Heuser (E.Ger) - training; style described in other film, dipping head when bar is at knees then throwing it back; works better if thrown up like Mitkov from Bulgaria and some of Poles; in this case it causes shoulders to go back instead of up

Bonk - training; notice flat feet during power position of pull, very good; in this case weight shift back is too much accentuated and he cannot come forward enough so jumps back, but in best lifts he does good job of getting weight transferred forward again

Wentzel - training; doing high pulls, bad because coming down to meet bar, throwing shoulders back, elbows going back; his training partner does better job of getting shoulders up and elbows up

Ciezki (E.Ger) - training; doing high pulls much better, getting elbows to lead up and shoulders going mostly up; East Germans said this assistance exercise is a must with shoulders going up and elbows leading up not back (although not all their lifters did it correctly); notice the big difference when elbows go up and when they go back

Bonk - training; doing high pulls; elbows go back instead of up, but does a lot of other things right; East Germans did a lot of heavy pulls close to the contest, much heavier than rest of countries, but it worked well for them

Todorov (Bulg) - training (in red shirt); elbows going back

Kuchev (Bulg) - training; squatting; doing high pulls with shoulders and elbows going back

Czechs - training (in yellow shirts); they do a lot of things right; notice good extension up; the one Czech doing high pulls shows about best elbows out to side and shoulders going up with elbows leading up and not coming down to meet bar too much

Hungarians - training (in white shirts and maroon pants); the one with blue shirt and maroon pants does the things we have discussed fairly well - hips high to start with, back angle maintained as bar gets to knees, shoulders go well in front of bar when bar at knees, good re-dip, good upward extension of shoulders and feet; throws head a little too far back when sometimes gets shoulders in back of bar and throws elbows out back so a little swing at top

Smalcerz (Pol) - training (in red and white warm-up); does good job in building momentum from floor to top; gets back a little too fast in rise so shoulders get in back of bar in power position; jumps too high with front foot in jerk (too much time in air)

Plachkov (Bulg) - warming up backstage (in blue shirt); does so many things correct but throws head back so winds up jumping back and sometimes swinging; shoulders go back

Alexeev (USSR) - warming up backstage (in all blue warm-up); notice great rise on toes that lighter men should copy

Plachkov - warming up backstage; jerking; gets front foot out quick because low to ground

Alexeev - warming up backstage; in the clean, again notice rise on toes, elbows to side, shoulders going up and chin in, re-dip is shallower than you would want, probably because he depends on his back more than many top flight lifters do

Plachkov - warming up; when he jerks really keeps rear in and throws knees forward in the dip; back leg should go farther back as does not hit full back position and sometimes buckles; back angle really drops on heavy cleans and he gets in trouble with swing and crashing (very evident on limit weights on competitive platform)

Czech superheavy - warming up; filmed to show the extra effort needed to do things correctly when joints are tight; although he does a lot of things right, his joints are tight and you can almost see the extra effort

TV that picks up movement of bar (like light attached to end of bar); instantaneous analysis (more on this in separate paper)

Alexeev - warming up; so efficient in jerk; low to ground in foot movement when moves fore and aft, goes so high on throw off chest

Bonk - in competition; he jumps up in the air, does not complete pull, and rushes down on drop under, wasting time getting underneath; his jerk is too high (too much wasted time in air when moving feet); really throws chest out front well; recovery with front foot too high (has lost heavy jerks by this and by recovering too fast)

Plachkov - in competition; back angle drops and back rounds; comes crashing down as swing is set up

This is an outline, a sketch; it is in no way complete. Some important points are: 1) In high pulls try to get elbows out to the side and leading up, extend upward with the shoulders, and do not go down to meet the bar. 2) In the jerk extend on toes in the drive and move feet close to ground when splitting. 3) Try for a wide split in the jerk by keeping close to ground; this allows a good wedge under the bar and permits a little bend in the back leg and also makes for a powerful 90° or obtuse angle when recovering from jerk (see other film).

1975 Moscow World Championships: Film #2

Won (Korea) - warming up (in blue warm-up); an Oriental using the double knee bend;

no swing; no frog style; form is good; flat foot when bar is in power position, which is good

Koral (USSR) - warming up (in blue warm-up); wide foot space; feet do not move; elbows under quick; no swing

Czarnecki (Pol) - warming up (in red and white warm-up); takes off too early and swings; shoulders go back

Kaczmarek (Pol) - warming up (in red and white warm-up); takes off too early and swings; shoulders go back

Kuchev (Bul) - warming up (in green top); elbows are to the side (good) and go up not back; in jerk wide, low split, not a leap; nice slide recovery

Kolesnikov (USSR) - warming up (in blue); takes off too early and swings

Koral - warming up; takes off too early, jumps back; jerk chest high; does not extend on toes, gets better during warm up

Kaczmarek - warming up; back too low in power position and therefore does not get as much hip and leg as should

Cameron (USA) - training; elbows to side (good); not deep enough scoop; good shoulder elevation; shoulders get in back of bar in power position on his miss; jumps and is in air too long

Wilhelm (USA) - training; scoop not deep enough; shoulders get a little in back of bar in power position; should explode more as bar goes up

Christov (Bul) - training (in green top); narrow foot stance at start and at end; gets elbows under quick; good flexibility in hips and thighs and ankles for narrow stance

Plachkov (Bul) - training (in blue top); throws head back and swings and jumps back

Christov - training; unique 1-2 exercise in split; low to ground split trajectory

Smalcerz (Pol) - training (in red and white warm-up); chest "forced through" in the jerk; feet flat in power position in clean (good); feet too high up in jerk

French lifters - training; stepping out well and chests high in jerk

Todorov (Bul) - training (in blue warm-up); takes off a little too early, shoulders go back and jumps back; gets better during training but in general goes too early; in clean not flat footed in power position (was in snatch) which causes loss of power; jerk slide recover nice and low to ground but should scrape toe more instead of heel

Jenson (Nor) - training; swings and jumps back; takes off too early

Bonk (E.Ger) - training; darn good; flat feet in power position; elbows go under good (no swing); like some lifters he starts with hips parallel but then he raises them quickly as bar comes off floor

Wentzel (E.Ger) - training; first rep takes off a little early and it crashes; flat foot in power position for pull; steps out good in jerk (notice obtuse angle)

Ciezki (E.Ger) - training (in maroon top); shoulders get in back of bar in power pull position and he jumps back; good flat foot in power position

Heuser (E.Ger) - training (in maroon top and blue shorts); head dip when bar gets to knee; swings head up fast but too far back and jumps back

Grippaldi (USA) - training; doing some jumps over broom stick

Nurikyen (Bul) - training; back comes up too fast and jumps back; gets better

Kirov (Bul) - training (in blue warm-up on far platform); gets shoulders a little in back of bar in power position in snatch but still extends up although leaning back

Todorov - training (in red shirt); pulls off heels and jumps back but transfers weight quick and compensates

Stoichev (Bul) - training (in red shirt); jerks okay but front foot goes too high and really does not "force chest through"

Kirov - training; example of starting with hips parallel in clean and then adjusting upward; gets better in jerk

Kuchev (Bul) - training (in green shirt); shoulders go in back of bar; good extension up but leans back; jerk gets chest and shoulders through, elbows up and out

Kirov - training; high pull; shoulders up but elbows back and he dips to meet bar (bad)

Grippaldi - training; doing pulls; back angle drops; does not let bar get high enough at crotch but uses his back and takes off too early

James (USA) - training (in white shirt); in snatch lets back come up a little too fast so shoulders are a little back and therefore jumps back; shoulder elevation is one of the best of any lifter

Kirov - warming up (in blue warm-up); re-dip not deep enough so starts early and jumps back; gets better during warm up but then repeats earlier mistakes

Nurikyan (Bul) - warming up (in blue warm-up); fairly good but jumps back; back angle lowers a little so swings a little

Kirov - warming up; same problems in clean but steps out better in jerk; moves his front foot too high in jerk recovery so swings a little

Milser (W.Ger) - training; doing power snatches to eye level and catching stiff knee and press out - good for getting elbows in under fast and also for remedial shoulder development; also notice good extension on toes

other West German - training; back comes up too quick; shoulders get in back of bar; swings

Mitkov (Bul) - training (in red shirt); rounds back; throws head back after bar reaches knees but does not swing back; this style like that of Poles is interesting; dip of head before swing not as pronounced; stays in power position with flat feet (good); jumps back but really gets push off, something like Rigert; maybe a little late in getting bodyweight back to front foot

Kuchev - training (in red shirt); power clean; low recovery with front foot in jerk (good)

Mitkov - training; leans forward on jerk; is tight in lower back, tries to get his chest high to compensate

Todorov - warming up; snatching; pulls off heels as comes off floor because hips too low but lets shoulders go well forward at knees so counterbalances

Kolesnikov - warming up; same as before - takes off too early and swings; jumps back

Todorov - warming up; clean good; not much jerk extension; cleans in good flat foot power position

Plachkov - training; jerk reaching up and out; getting leg out (notice front angle is obtuse) in jerk; recovery a little high but gets better as days progress

Mitkov - warming up; much as before; really gets hips back in jerk (loses some out front

Heckel (Czech) - warming up; split fairly good although shoulders probably going back because he does not re-dip enough; goes on toes too early (see right foot) so swings some; like Mitkov front foot leaves way too early on jerk

Kolev (Bul) - warming up; hips start low and then go high on clean from floor; dip not deep; jerk does not get out front enough (he has lost a lot)

Christov - training; narrow stance when starts and ends in snatch; must be very flexible in hips and ankles to do this; in jerk gets front foot out very quick and at 90° angle

Shary (USSR) - warming up (in blue warm-up); very good clean; re-dip not as low as could be but good coordination over-all; really reaches front foot out; chest high; incomplete jerk very common when warming up; notice he leans back when going into jerk (not afraid to go for it!)

198 lb. Australian - warming up; notice wide stance, so wide seems to limit reentry; elbows pointed back; never gets weight back on front foot when re-dips and bar leaves center of gravilty around hips

Greek - warming up; rounded back; takes off too early; shoulders go back and swings; head dips around knees - influence of Polish coach

Hungarian - warming up; hips way too low; does not adjust; head too far up at start

Polterosky (USSR) - warming up (in red shirt, blue sweats); does a lot of things right

Hungarian - warming up; head goes back too far; throws shoulders too far back

East German - warming up; not bad except seems like toes pointed out too much with
    narrow stance; goes on toes too early; lack of stability so takes off early;
    if he waited could push off flat footed

    Again, this is an outline, a sketch to help viewers; it is in no way complete.
Some important points are: 1) Flat foot when in power pull position is important.
2) Step out with front foot in jerk so you get at least a 90° angle and maybe an
obtuse angle; you want a wide split, and going into it you should be low to the
ground). 3) Shoulders should be in front of bar in the power position so you do
not lean back. 4) The deeper the re-dip, the more power from legs and hips. 5) A
dip of the head when the bar is at the knees and then throwing it back is being
tried for more extension by some lifters; this is new and hard to coordinate.

SECTION III

TRAINING METHODS

1

Fast Twitch and Slow Twitch Muscle Fibers
and
Some of Their Meanings to Olympic Weightlifters and Coaches

Muscle fiber is made up of fast twitch (FT) and slow twitch (ST) muscle fibers. FT muscle fibers account for the fast movements of a muscle; they tire quickly. ST muscle fibers contract slower but they do not tire easily. A good sprinter will have over 80% FT and less than 20% ST muscle fibers. A good marathon runner will have over 70% ST and less than 30% FT muscle fibers. We could expect a good weight- lifter to be like a sprinter. A good sprinter will have a vertical jump of over 25 inches. A good marathon runner will have a vertical jump of under 20 inches. Paul Anderson had a vertical jump of 31 inches (highest ever recorded). Alexeev has a vertical jump of 30 inches. Both of these men weighed over 350 pounds when tested. One can expect that some of the great weightlifting champions in catego- ries under super heavy who do not have excess weight would have vertical jumps over 31 inches, but nobody has tested them.

Nothing can be done through training to change one's proportion of FT and ST fibers since each has a different nerve supply. However, within the FT fibers there is room for change through training. This is because there are red fibers which are FT and white fibers which are FT. The red fibers are slower than the white FT fibers. This difference within the FT fibers is called quality. The FT fibers either have the quality of red fibers or the quality of white fibers.

The interchanging of the red and white FT fibers depends on the type of train- ing the fibers undergo and upon sex hormone activity. Slow movement training will have the effect of converting some of the white FT fibers into red FT fibers. Fast movement training will have the effect of converting some of the red FT fibers into white FT fibers.

Slow movement training is comprised of movements during which the athlete is not going as fast as he could. Even if he is going against a tremendous weight, say a clean or snatch dead lift of upward of 125% of what he can clean or snatch, he will be training more FT fibers if he thinks speed (while maintaining good form). In fact, such deep penetrating exercises as isokinetics, functional isometrics, electrostimulation, dead stops, and eccentric contraction, if the athlete is think- ing speed and maintaining good form, are some of the advanced ways of activating FT fibers which were previously dormant. They will be activated as red (slower) FT fibers but can later be trained to become white (faster) FT fibers. It is of ut- most importance that the athlete think speed. If he does not, he will be activat- ing more dormant ST fibers because ST and FT muscle fibers each have their own nerve supply.

Because of the recent finding of distinct nerve supply between the ST and FT fibers and later talks with world leaders in our sport, I must add to statements I made in Bulgaria #5 (Peaking in Terms of Reps) and Marseille-Moscow #2 (Leg Work). I said that high reps can increase power because after the slow twitch fibers are exhausted from the increase in reps, the fast twitch fibers are brought into play. Apparently this takes place as long as the lifter thinks speed after he starts be- coming exhausted. FT fibers will be activated and trained as red FT fibers. Later they can be converted to white FT fibers.

Exactly how the ST and FT muscle fibers work together in such movements as the snatch or clean and jerk, which begin slow and end fast, is not clear. Many medical people associated with our sport across the world believe that the ST fibers help the FT fibers overcome the weight at the beginning but stop functioning as the movement becomes too fast for them to contribute any force.

This knowledge has many practical training implications, three of which I would like to discuss. One, training should include pulling heavy weights off the floor or squatting with heavy weights at near bottom and a little above parallel in order to activate both FT and ST fibers since both are needed to overcome the inertia of the weight or bad leverage position. Thinking normally will activate more ST fibers and thinking speed will activate more FT fibers. Since the belief is now that the lifter should pull or rise as fast as possible with coordination (without breaking good form), the lifter should think speed when doing pulls or squats as described above. This way the fibers in the proportion used in the actual snatch or clean and jerk and rising from the clean would be activated.

Two, using heavy weights in the above manner and using deep penetrating exercises (such as isokinetics, functional isometrics, electrostimulation, dead stops, eccentric contraction and high rep squats), because the movement is slow, activates the FT fibers which are predominantly red. Since more white fibers are needed because the snatch and clean and jerk are done at faster speeds, it is necessary to train the newly activated red FT fibers at the athletic speed that will be needed to do the snatch and clean and jerk. Therefore, the spacing of slow movements (even though done thinking fast) with the fast movements should be carefully determined. And that is what is empirically stated in what I wrote about percentages in such articles as Bulgaria #3 (Training Programs), Bulgaria #5 (Peaking in Terms of Reps), Marseille-Moscow #2 (Leg Work) and Specificity of Speed. Within these articles are guidelines of percentages to use at what intervals whether it be in pulling, leg work, overhead work, and so on. These are guidelines that have been drawn up based on the successful programs of the top weightlifting nations.

Three, a device is needed to measure the speed of movement of the bar in order to: 1) find out what the speed of the bar is at near maximum and maximum snatch and clean and jerk and 2) train at that athletic speed when training either in the snatch and clean and jerk or the assistant exercises. This type of measurement device is being used in Bulgaria, the Soviet Union, East Germany and possibly in Poland.

Simply, this all boils down to activating the appropriate muscle fibers and then training them at the speed of the snatch and clean and jerk.

2

Training Methods - Bulgaria #3

In the first two articles I wrote upon my return from Bulgaria I said that we can produce international stars in lifting; it is within our capability to do so. What is so different from our swimmers training four hours a day and going to school or work and a lifter doing the same? I also said not everybody would want to do this or could but some would and could. And to get the ones that could, we need to be more cognizant of the process of selection. I included simple meaningful tests to use as a means of selecting prospective good lifters.

Now I want to say that although we are on the right track in our training methods, there are some things that should be stressed even more, and there are some things which should be thought of in a different manner. What this amounts to is organizing and putting to work some of the great ideas born out by practical results in the weightlifting field. What I am going to relate should be viewed in a certain perspective. One, it cannot be fully explained in something as short as this paper. That is why I am urging more clinics, for both coaches and athletes. There are intangibles which are difficult to put into writing unless time is allotted to write a book (this should be done but until it is done we have to get out the information as fast as possible and in as meaningful a way as possible). Two, this is not a pure Bulgarian system or any other system because we are Americans and live in different conditions. It is a system that I believe can be the most meaningful to Americans. I find the Bulgarian system the most applicable because of its sound technical base, success and its similarity to what we could do in this country, even though the Bulgarian lifters are state supported.

The Meaning of Training Phases

It should be evident to even the most novice athlete that to get in top shape he conditions himself for a contest and then he competes in a contest. After a while he may become stale and performance drops off. Now this has a very real physiological basis depending in part on what is happening in the adrenal glands. Hans Selye, famed Canadian research doctor, has on many occasions explained his theory of stress by three stages: 1) An alarm stage which is the phase of adaptation during which training is initiated and progress is made toward peak performance. This can be from 4 to 12 weeks. 2) A resistance stage which is the complete adaptation or achievement of peak condition which lasts 3 to 6 weeks. 3) An exhaustion stage which is readaptation to the loss of peak condition.

This means that a preliminary phase, a contest phase and a post contest or readaptation phase for lifting are real, not imaginary; there are certain boundaries of time for getting ready for competition, reaching and maintaining the peak for the competition and readapting again for the next competition. It becomes even more meaningful the higher a lifter travels up the scale in competition because the stresses are more.

Let us use as an example the elite lifter. For him this whole preliminary contest and readaptation cycle takes 16 weeks. This can be divided into an 8 week preparation phase, a 6 week contest phase and a 2 week readaptation phase. This works out to three peaks (three 16 week periods) per year with a 4 week period of vacation.

The class four lifter cannot fit exactly into the stress theory because he is new. He will make good progress because he is new and not wholly because of the correct program he is on. However, it is applicable to him because if he is to progress he needs a meaningful structure to train by so that he will make the most progress possible. He must learn a correct training system so when he does progress and changes categories, he will have trained under a system which will bring out continued progress in him. There is no reason for many of our lifters to get bogged down in their categories. If they trained under a sound system their bodies could be coaxed into far more progress.

Below are listed the cycles of competitions and the length of training phases for our different classes (categories).

Class IV

Eight competitions every 5 to 6 weeks. Two phases of four competitions with a vacation between each phase.

#1	#2	#3	#4
1-2 wk prep.	1-2 wk prep.	1-2 wk prep.	1-2 wk prep.
3 wk contest	3 wk contest	3 wk contest	3 wk contest
1 wk readapt	1 wk readapt	1 wk readapt	1 wk readapt

around 24 weeks total depending on selection

vacation

#5	#6	#7	#8
same as #1	same as #2	same as #3	same as #4

Class III

Six competitions every 7 to 8 weeks. Two phases of three competitions with a vacation between each phase.

#1	#2	#3
3 wk prep	2-3 wk prep	2-3 wk prep
4 wk contest	4 wk contest	4 wk contest
1 wk readapt	1 wk readapt	1 wk readapt

around 23 weeks total depending on selection

vacation

#4	#5	#6
same as #1	same as #2	same as #3

Class II

Five competitions every 9 to 10 weeks. One phase of five competitions with a vacation at the end.

#1	#2	#3	#4	#5
5 wk prep	5 wk prep	5 wk prep	5 wk prep	5 wk prep
4 wk contest	4 wk contest	4 wk contest	4 wk contest	4 wk contest
1 wk readapt	1 wk readapt	1 wk readapt	1 wk readapt	1 wk readapt

Class I

Four competitions every 12 weeks in one phase with a vacation at the end.

#1	#2	#3	#4
6 wk prep	6 wk prep	6 wk prep	6 wk prep
5 wk contest	5 wk contest	5 wk contest	5 wk contest
1 wk readapt	1 wk readapt	1 wk readapt	1 wk readapt

<u>Master and Elite</u>
Three competitions every 16 weeks in one phase with a vacation at the end.

#1	#2	#3
8 wk prep	8 wk prep	8 wk prep
6 wk contest	6 wk contest	6 wk contest
2 wk readapt	2 wk readapt	2 wk readapt

It is recognized and understood that our contests in the United States will not allow this to be followed exactly, but they come fairly close. And if something is off a few weeks, adaptation will have to be made. However, this guideline is also set up to try to guide our meet directors in the placement of their meets. This means having contests scheduled by classes (categories) where possible. Some places are already doing this. This also means having more local support financially so our lifters can travel when need be to closely follow such a training cycle.

It is also recognized that other contests will come up during this time in which a lifter may want to lift for a variety of reasons. This is fine, but he should treat these contests as workouts and not peak for them. He may train on the same day after this type of contest is over with; this is very prevalent in other countries. Sometimes entering such a contest will catch a lifter unexpectedly at his best; in this case he should not hold back. The important thing is to have treated the contest as a workout by not peaking for it. If the weights feel extra light in such a contest, the lifter may go for records.

The number of competitions for lower category lifters is more than the number for lifters in higher categories. This is extremely important for development. It must be stressed that what happens in the gym is only part of the development. The lifter must get used to and even thrive on competition. There is so much to learn from competition that the many peaks for a lower category lifter are important if he is to develop fully and eventually lift the most he possibly could at the end of his lifting career. The higher category lifter has had many competitions in the past and no longer needs as many. He is now a veteran and he needs to spend more time on making his body respond to higher training intensities.

The Preparation Phase

The preparation phase brings the body to the point where it is able to go into peak phase and maintain it. It is important to know that in this phase much of the time the lifter is lifting while tired. He trains to a tired point and then trains more. He is actually doing more work at higher intensity than during the phase that follows which is the contest phase. This idea of training while tired during the preparation period is a concept developed by the Bulgarians to good success, but it is not limited to weightlifting. Such sports as track and field and swimming have used it for years.

When I say the lifter is doing more work during the preparation phase, I mean actual _time_ training. This time concept was also developed by the Bulgarians. They recognized that work as measured by existing tonnage measurements was grossly in error, so why add it up. This is something I have pointed out in past clinics, based on my experience in Japan, and I was glad to see it confirmed by the Bulgarians; they have not used the tonnage system for years. What they measure is time spent per type of exercise per lifting rating (class). It is taken for granted that a lifter will rest two to three minutes between lifts. This is also a way of scheduling workouts which other sports such as football and basketball have used with success. It means scheduling time for drills in accordance with each drill's importance to the final result so that each workout is as productive as possible.

51

Contest Phase

The contest phase starts when the lifter wants to go into peak condition and hold it for the competition. The time allotted to training is reduced; the lifter trains till he is tired and then no more. Workouts are more short and sweet. On paper they may not seem that much shorter, but it is that little bit of a slack off in work which allows a freshness on the part of the lifter. If there is too much slack off, the lifter loses the edge he is building for.

The Readaptation Phase

The readaptation phase is one of coming down off of a peak, maintaining good weightlifting physical condition, and easing into another cycle of preparation. This is a very important phase. I have already stated that the body needs this to recuperate. The adrenals have been at a hyperactive stage for weeks, and they cannot take any further output. The mental, physical and emotional stress of preparation and then competition leads to a state of exhaustion. If a lifter goes from a contest immediately back into a preparation phase, he is not allowing the adrenals to recuperate. After 7 to 18 weeks the adrenals require a period of recuperation. If they do not get it, not only is their output not returned to normal but also there is a drop in the eosinophil count (one of the white blood cells) because of too much constant physical, mental and emotional stress.

Vacation

A vacation should really be called active rest. A complete change of living habits (without going against health) should take place in order for the lifter to feel fresh for the upcoming training sessions. The theory is to have fun actively. It is taken for granted that athletes like movement; therefore, when they go on vacation they should have fun with movement. This way they enjoy themselves, a change of pace is attained, and their general physical condition does not deteriorate. Sports suggested for a vacation are: basketball, soccer, track and field, paddleball, handball, volleyball, gymnastics, swimming, bicycling, skiing and iceskating. The lifter can engage in these sports in his own town or wherever he goes. He should have fun with them and just enjoy the movement of activity, letting his mind and emotions rest.

Practical and Realistic Training Time for Progress

The Bulgarians train longer than the amount of time presented here. I have adapted their training time to something realistic for us. Even so, to some lifters it will seem too long. If so, maybe such lifters are overachieving for their class; their bodies are just not adaptable to such training. Such a lifter might try training one category less than his actual rating. But remember, to lift more weight, the lifter must wisely increase his intensity and the amount of work. There might be a stage he will reach wherein his body goes down hill. But with systematic training and excellent health habits the lifter can probably adapt to more intensity and work. The theory of adaptability is the key to getting the most out of the body. We have only to look at the long intense training sessions (4-6 hours) of our top swimmers and wrestlers to know this can be done. They did not start out with such lengthy sessions, but they followed adaptive training methods of increasing work and intensity, and when their bodies adapted, they swam faster and wrestled better.

There will be casualties along the way. One lifter's body will be able to produce less; another's will produce more. That is one reason why there are so few world champions. It is nothing that can be helped and nothing personally against a lifter. It is also a reason why our selection process should be good so that we can get lifters with the physical constitution that can adapt to the high levels of stress needed to progress.

In any case, each lifter should give himself every chance of success. I have already mentioned the necessity of excellent health habits. If a lifter does not follow excellent health habits, his body cannot adapt as well to increasing stress. This means regular sleeping habits. It means eating good. It means no smoking. This also means being very careful of alcohol. A few beers once in a while is not going to hurt a lifter, but any more is going to have a pronounced effect on his recovery from workouts. Alcohol affects the enzymatic system which plays such an important role in assimilation of foods. Such health habits also include the lifter being at peace with himself. There will be enough emotional stress just training and competing; to add to it other outside problems means the lifter cannot recover well enough between workouts.

I hope the idea of discipline has come across. This was stressed at the European Coaches' Conference time and time again, not only by the Bulgarians but also by the other countries. Even the Russians said the key to the Bulgarian success is discipline. Such intense training cannot be done without it. This word takes in so much. Many training problems are solved just by having discipline.

Preparation Phase	Elite	Master	I	II	III	IV
hours each workout	3-3½	2½-3	2-2½	1¾-2	1½-1¾	1¼-1½
hours per week	15-17½	12½-15	10-12½	8¾-10	6-7	3¾-4½
training sessions/week	5	5	5	5	4	3

Contest Phase						
hours each workout	2½-3	2-2½	1½-1¾	1¼-1½	1-1¼	1-1¼
hours per week	12½-15	10-12½	7½-8¾	6¼-7½	4-6	3-3¾
training sessions/week	5	5	5	5	4	3

Readaptation Phase						
hours each workout	1½-1¾	1½	1¼-1½	1-1¼	¾-1	½-¾
hours per week	7½-8¾	7½	6¼-7½	5-6¼	3-4	1½-2¼
training sessions/week	5	5	5	5	4	3

Vacation						
hours each fun period	1	1	1	1	1	1
fun periods per week	5	5	5	4	3	3

Related Exercises

To help organize the countless number of exercises, we group related ones. Each one can be designated as technique oriented, power oriented or both. Below are such listings.

Snatch Related	Technique/Power	Jerk Related	Technique/Power
1. Complete from floor	T	1. Push press	P
2. From knees	T	2. Push up and out	P
3. From mid-thigh	T	3. On toes, split & recover	T or P
4. Dead lift to knees	T or P	4. Push drive	P
5. Power snatch	P	5. Balance	T
6. High pull – straight arms	T or P	6. Jerk – eyes closed	T
7. High pull – arms coming up	T or P	7. Front squat and jerk	T
8. Overhead squat	T	8. Jerk from rack	T
9. Isokinetics	P	9. Isokinetics	P
10. Eccentric contraction	P	10. Eccentric contraction	P

Clean Related	Technique/Power	Leg Related	Technique/Power
1. Complete from floor	T	1. Front squat	P
2. From knees	T	2. Super killer squat	P
3. From mid-thigh	T	3. Speed squat	P
4. Dead lift to knees	T or P	4. Pre-exhaustion	P
5. Power clean	P	5. Back squat (Olympic)	P
6. High pull - straight arms	T or P	6. Back squat (pull position)	T or P
7. High pull - arms coming up	T or P	7. Split squat	P
8. Position squat	T	8. Olympic clean dead lift	T or P
9. Isokinetics	P	9. Isokinetics	P
10. Eccentric contraction	P	10. Eccentric contraction	P

Remedial Exercises

Leg	Back	Shoulder
1. Leg extension	1. Good morning	1. Seat press
2. Leg curl	2. Hyperextension	2. Bench press
3. Leg push	3. Stiff leg dead lift	3. Behind neck press
4. Hack machine	4. Three fourths hyperextension	4. Stand military press
5. Isokinetics	5. Isokinetics	5. Power snatch to forehead and press out
	6. Bent knee sit-ups	

Exercise Groupings

Exercises are grouped into categories according to specific goals of a workout and then these categories are practiced so many times per week depending on the rating (class) of the lifter. Below are listed these categories and the number of times per week they are practiced.

Class	Sn Tech	Sn Pw	C&J Tech	Cl Tech	Cl Pw	Jk Pw	Jk Tech	Leg	Remedial Leg	Back	Shldr	TOTAL
#IV & below	2	1	2	1	1	2	1	2	1	1	1	15
#III	2	2	2	1	2	2	1	2	1	2	2	19
#II	2	2	2	1	2	3	2	3	2	2	2	23
#I	3	3	2	1	3	4	2	3	2	2	2	27
Master	3	4	2	1	4	5	2	4	2	2	2	31
Elite	3	5	2	1	5	6	2	5	2	2	2	35

Some of the thoughts behind the above are: 1) As the lifter advances in rating and style is learned, strength must be emphasized more. 2) The clean and jerk is separated for some specialized learning since it is made up of two separate skills, but then it is practiced in its entirety. 3) There is a progression in the number of times various facets are practiced per week. 4) Remedial exercises play a part in the program.

Let me define remedial exercises. These are exercises which should give specialized strengthening around the back, leg and shoulder joints. They are not practiced for very long nor are they emphasized in intensity. To place more emphasis on them might open a lifter up to injury or overdevelopment; he does not want to get injured doing the exercises. Part of the purpose of such exercises is to balance possible overdevelopment incurred when doing the standard exercises. Leg curls would be such an exercise to balance the development of the quads. Bench presses would be another to balance pulls. We do not need big pecs and we do not need to be able to bench big weights, but we do want strength in the chest area for the reason stated above and for general shoulder area conditioning. Seated presses do not help the first part of the jerk, but by strengthening that area they could prevent an injury there. Just a few sets into the time allotted at the end of a time period with

80-90% of the best for those reps engaged in (for example, 80% of best for 5 reps) would be sufficient for the remedial exercises.

Actual Practice Layout

Listed below for each class is a layout of the number of times exercise grouped categories are practiced each week and the time allotted per workout for the exercises. The exercises can be inserted. Technique groups are placed during the practice at the time that the lifter would be most fresh. Remedial exercises are at the end of the practices. The explanation of warm-ups and games and recovery will be presented after these practice layouts.

Elite

	Day #1	Day #2	Day #3	Day #4	Day #5
a.m.	1. Sn Tech	1. C&J Tech	1. Jk Tech	1. C&J Tech	1. Leg
	2. Sn Pw	2. Cl Pw	2. Cl Pw	2. Sn Tech	2. Jk Pw
	3. Jk Pw	3. Jk Pw	3. Jk Pw	3. Jk Pw	3. Sn Pw
p.m.	4. Jk Tech	4. Sn Tech	4. Leg	4. Cl Pw	4. Cl Tech
	5. Sn Pw	5. Sn Pw	5. Sn Pw	5. Leg	5. Jk Pw
	6. Leg	6. Cl Pw	6. Shldr Remed	6. Leg Remed	6. Cl Pw
	7. Shldr Remed	7. Leg Remed	7. Bk Remed	7. Bk Remed	7. Leg

Time Allotted	Prep Period (in minutes)	Contest Period (in minutes)	Readaptability Period (in minutes)
1. Snatch Tech, Clean & Jerk Tech	35	30	20
2. Snatch Power, Clean Power	20-25	20-25	15
3. Jerk Tech & Power, Clean Tech	20	15	5-7
4. Leg	25-30	20-25	15
5. Remedials	15	10	5-7
6. Warm-ups	15	15	10
7. Games	40	20	25
Approximate Total	3 hours	2¾ hours	1½-1¾ hours

Master

	Day #1	Day #2	Day #3	Day #4	Day #5
a.m.	1. Sn Tech	1. C&J Tech	1. Jk Tech	1. C&J Tech	1. Leg
	2. Sn Pw	2. Cl Pw	2. Jk Pw	2. Sn Tech	2. Jk Pw
	3. Jk Pw	3. Jk Pw	3. Sn Pw	3. Jk Pw	3. Sn Pw
p.m.	4. Jk Tech	4. Sn Tech	4. Leg	4. Cl Pw	4. Cl Tech
	5. Leg	5. Sn Pw	5. Shldr Remed	5. Leg	5. Cl Pw
	6. Bk Remed	6. Cl Pw	6. Bk Remed	6. Leg Remed	6. Shldr Rem
		7. Leg Remed			

Time Allotted	Prep Period (in minutes)	Contest Period (in minutes)	Readaptability Period (in minutes)
1. Snatch Tech, Clean & Jerk Tech	30-35	25-30	15-20
2. Snatch Power, Clean Power	20-25	20-25	15
3. Jerk Tech & Power, Clean Tech	15	15	5
4. Leg	20-25	15-20	15
5. Remedials	10	10	5-7
6. Warm-ups	15	15	10
7. Games	40	20	20
Approximate Total	2½-2¾ hours	2-2¼ hours	1½ hours

Class I

Day #1	Day #2	Day #3	Day #4	Day #5
1. Sn Tech	1. C&J Tech	1. Jk Tech	1. C&J Tech	1. Cl Tech
2. Sn Pw	2. Sn Tech	2. Jk Pw	2. Sn Tech	2. Leg
3. Jk Tech	3. Cl Pw	3. Sn Pw	3. Jk Pw	3. Jk Pw
4. Leg	4. Jk Pw	4. Leg	4. Cl Pw	4. Sn Pw
5. Bk Remed	5. Leg Remed	5. Shldr Remed	5. Leg Remed	5. Cl Pw
		6. Bk Remed		6. Shldr Remed

Time Allotted	Prep Period (in minutes)	Contest Period (in minutes)	Readaptability Period (in minutes)
1. Snatch Tech, Clean & Jerk Tech	25-30	20-25	15
2. Snatch Power, Clean Power	20	20	12
3. Jerk Tech & Power, Clean Tech	15	15	5
4. Leg	20	15	12
5. Remedials	10	10	5-7
6. Warm-ups	15	15	10
7. Games	30	15	15
Approximate Total	2¼ hours	1¾-2 hours	1¼ hours

Class II

Day #1	Day #2	Day #3	Day #4	Day #5
1. Sn Tech	1. C&J Tech	1. Jk Tech	1. C&J Tech	1. Cl Tech
2. Sn Pw	2. Cl Pw	2. Leg	2. Sn Tech	2. Jk Pw
3. Jk Tech	3. Jk Pw	3. Shldr Remed	3. Jk Pw	3. Leg
4. Leg	4. Leg Remed	4. Bk Remed	4. Cl Pw	4. Sn Pw
5. Bk Remed			5. Leg Remed	5. Shldr Remed

Time Allotted	Prep Period (in minutes)	Contest Period (in minutes)	Readaptability Period (in minutes)
1. Snatch Tech, Clean & Jerk Tech	20-25	20	12
2. Snatch Power, Clean Power	15	15	10
3. Jerk Tech & Power, Clean Tech	15	10	5
4. Leg	15	12-15	10
5. Remedials	10	10	5-7
6. Warm-ups	10	10	10
7. Games	25	15	15
Approximate Total	1¾-2 hours	1¼ hours	1-1¼ hours

Class III

Day #1	Day #2	Day #3	Day #4
1. Sn Tech	1. C&J Tech	1. Jk Tech	1. C&J Tech
2. Cl Tech	2. Jk Pw	2. Sn Tech	2. Jk Pw
3. Cl Pw	3. Sn Pw	3. Cl Pw	3. Sn Pw
4. Leg	4. Leg Remed	4. Leg	4. Bk Remed
5. Shldr Remed	5. Bk Remed	5. Shldr Remed	

Time Allotted	Prep Period (in minutes)	Contest Period (in minutes)	Readaptability Period (in minutes)
1. Snatch Tech, Clean & Jerk Tech	15-20	15	10
2. Snatch Power, Clean Power	12-15	12	8
3. Jerk Tech & Power, Clean Tech	10	10	5
4. Leg	12-15	12	8
5. Remedials	10	10	5
6. Warm-ups	10	10	10
7. Games	20	15	10
Approximate Total	1½-1¾ hours	1½ hours	1 hour

Class IV

Day #1	Day #2	Day #3
1. Sn Tech	1. C&J Tech	1. C&J Tech
2. Cl Tech	2. Cl Pw	2. Sn Tech
3. Jk Pw	3. Jk Tech	3. Sn Pw
4. Leg	4. Jk Pw	4. Leg
5. Bk Remed	5. Leg Remed	5. Shldr Remed

Time Allotted	Prep Period (in minutes)	Contest Period (in minutes)	Readaptability Period (in minutes)
1. Snatch Tech, Clean & Jerk Tech	15	15	5
2. Snatch Power, Clean Power	12-15	12	5
3. Jerk Tech & Power, Clean Tech	10	10	5
4. Leg	12-15	10	5
5. Remedials	5	5	5
6. Warm-ups	10	10	10
7. Games	15	10	10
Approximate Total	1¼-1½ hours	1¼ hours	45 minutes

There are two methods of doing the exercises which fit into the time allotted per exercise grouping in the Readaptability Period. One method is for the lifter to choose a weight that is within 50-60% of his best and do four to six repetitions, doing as many sets as the time allotted calls for, resting only one minute between sets. A second method is for the lifter to choose a weight that is within 40-50% of his best and do four to six repetitions, going from exercise to exercise with no rest and repeating the exercises in a circuit. The exercises can be grouped so that the time allotted to exercise related grouping is covered and the exercises are placed so they do not fatigue any one muscle group, something like the old PHA system of the mid and late 1960's.

As was stated earlier, the readaptation phase is one of coming down off a peak, maintaining good weightlifting physical condition and easing into another cycle of preparation. The adrenal glands are given a chance to rest and recuperate. In either of the two methods described above, all this can be accomplished because coordinated movements are being performed without emotional stress. It is enough of a change of pace to be refreshing and enough fast work to be physically stimulating. At the end of this phase or period the lifter is in shape mentally, physically and emotionally to go into the preparation phase of the next cycle.

Warming-up

The warm-up should be well planned, organized and goal oriented. It is the warm-up which not only prevents both micro and major injuries but also sets the mood for the workout. A lifter can feel varying degrees of enthusiasm going into a workout; if he goes through a well designed warm-up his enthusiasm will rise.

Improved circulation is one goal of warming-up. There are circulatory adjustments the cardiovascular system makes in order to handle increased activity. Circulation should be increased throughout the whole muscular frame.

Specific flexibility is another goal. A warm-up must increase the flexibility in areas most useful to the lifter.

Specific coordination patterns used in lifting should be a third goal of warming up. Extemporaneous movement patterns during the warm-up, while increasing circulation, do nothing for adding more practice of movement patterns along the lines a lifter can use.

To reach the goals of increased circulation, specific flexibility and specific coordination, the warm-up is best designed in a circuit with exercises placed in the circuit. A circuit has these advantages: 1) It can be performed in a small place. 2) It offers an organized pattern which is a goal itself and thus more meaningful than just warming-up haphazardly. 3) It offers a method of organization of warm-up exercises which stimulates the desire to train and which does not tire out the lifter.

With the above in mind, here is an example of how a circuit can be designed.

Start:

(1) Ankle Stretch
(2) 20 high steps forward ⟶ (3) Split Squat

(5) Scapula Raise ⟵ (4) 50 high steps backward
(6) Wrist Stretch

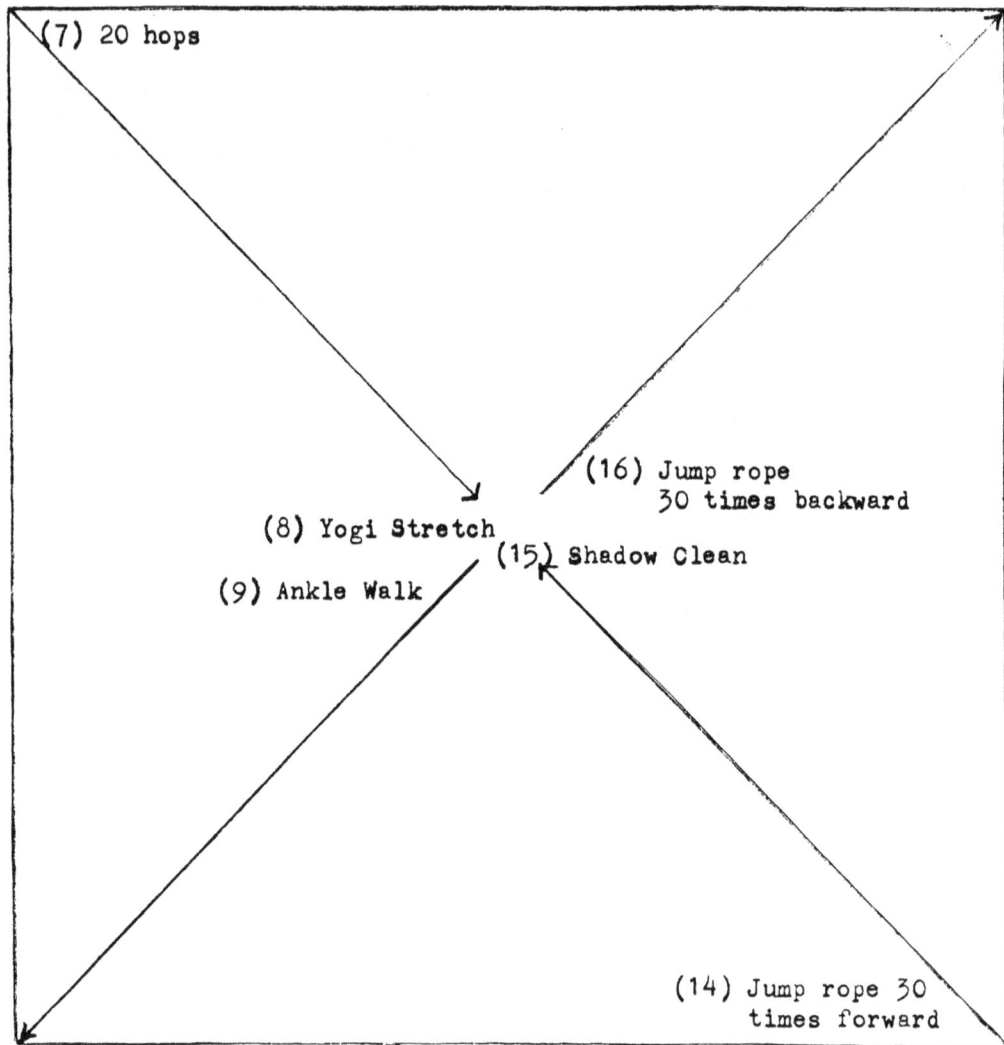

(17) Shadow Snatch

(7) 20 hops

(16) Jump rope
30 times backward

(8) Yogi Stretch   (15) Shadow Clean

(9) Ankle Walk

(14) Jump rope 30
times forward

(10) Arm Circle   (13) Shadow Jerk
(11) Crab Walk ⟶ (12) Dislocates

The lifter should go through this circuit as many times as it takes to complete a 10-15 minute warm-up. He does the exercise as correctly as possible but also as fast as possible. The lifter is only in competition against himself so it is a race with himself and nobody else.

Three types of exercises were chosen and placed in order that: 1) they will invigorate the lifter, 2) gradual loosening will take place before complicated movements are performed, and 3) maximum use can be made of a small room. While there are other exercises which can be substituted for the ones presented, the jerk, clean and snatch shadow movements should be included in any type of circuit warm-up. The following is a brief explanation of the exercises used.

Flexibility Exercises

1. Ankle Walk - Bend over, grasp back of heels and walk. This stretches the hamstrings.
2. Ankle Stretch - Lean on a solid surface (arms outstretched, palms against the surface) and put one foot as far back as you can, keeping the whole foot flat on the floor. When you get to the point where the heel starts to come up, then stretch it down by pushing down and back on that foot. Push down for 3 to 5 seconds, relax and follow with two to four more bouts of 3 to 5 seconds. Then do the same with the other foot.
3. Yogi Crotch Stretch - Sit down, bend the knees and put the soles of the feet together, bringing the feet as close to the crotch as possible. Grab ankles with hands, arms between thighs, and put elbows on thighs, using them and the forearms as levers to push down and out on the thighs. This will stretch the adductors (inside of thighs). Hold the maximum stretch for 3 to 5 seconds and do the stretch 2 to 4 times.
4. Arm Circle - Hold arms out to the side. Make 10 small firm circles forward and then 10 small firm circles backward.
5. Dislocates - Take a broom stick and using the snatch grip move the stick from overhead to behind the head and down to the lower back. Return the stick to the overhead position. Repeat 10 times.
6. Scapula Raise - Stand with hands on two chairs shoulder distance apart or with hands on parallel bars. Completely relax the scapula and lean down on the hands letting the shoulders come up to the ears. Hold for 3 to 5 seconds and then drop the shoulders. Repeat 2 to 4 times.
7. Wrist Stretch - Stand arm distance away from a wall. Extend one arm putting the palm on the wall, fingers pointing down. Move the palm up the wall until it will not stay flat on the wall. Then lean into the wall so the palm does touch it again. Hold for 3 to 5 seconds and repeat 2 to 4 times. Do both wrists.
8. Split Squat - Put one foot in front and the other in back like a split clean or snatch. Put hands overhead and drop down into a low split keeping the trunk erect. Stay in this low position 3 to 5 seconds and repeat 2 to 4 times. Let your bodyweight push you down far. Work both legs.

Coordination Exercises

Shadow Jerk, Shadow Clean and Shadow Snatch - For each of these go through the exercise like you normally would with a bar. Concentrate on hitting all positions as you go through the movement. Try to make the movement fluid as you do it for 5 repetitions. Because no weight is present you will feel clumsy to begin with, but this will subside if you go through the exercise purposefully and slowly, striving for a fluid motion. With each repetition pick up the tempo.

Circulatory Exercises

1. Crab Walk - Sit on the floor and put palms on floor a little behind the shoul-

ders with the fingers pointing back. The feet are out front with the knees bent. Raise the rear end off the floor and on all fours walk backward, one arm and the opposite leg going back together.

2. Jump Rope - Jump using any of a variety of steps you might know. Take 30 jumps to reach your destination. This way height of jump is emphasized and not ground covered.

3. Hops - The distance is short for 20 hops, which is good because you want to concentrate more on height than distance. Extend the knees, hips, back and feet fully as you hop.

Games

Games are used in the workout schedule for some very good reasons. The most obvious is to gain some cardiovascular strength. Anybody who says weightlifting is not an endurance sport does not understand that to keep your adrenaline up for the many hours of competition takes real endurance. If the cardiovascular system is developed, then stamina can be called on late in the contest because a lot of blood is not only being pumped through the system but is also being tapped by the cells. This means more oxygen and nutrients go to the cells and more toxins are gotten rid of.

A second reason for games is to reinforce movement patterns that are similar to those used in weightlifting and that are power oriented. This is why, for example, volleyball and basketball should be played a lot. If you have ever played a good game of either, you know how much your legs and hips get worked. Of course broad jumping, high jumping and shot putting are good to "play" because of power movement patterns similar to lifting.

A third reason for games is to develop competitiveness. Although competitiveness is natural to man, it is not always brought out or reinforced, so it never gets developed to its full potential. Not even a class four lifter competes in very many competitions each year. This is why, for one reason, many lifters are gym lifters. They never had much training in competitiveness as they were developing. By playing games in the training routine and placing emphasis on beating the next man's mark or beating the other team, competitiveness is developed. This can be a lot of fun, by mixing up what type of competitions (e.g. tournaments) you will have and even inventing a few.

Change of pace is a fourth reason for including games in your workout schedule. The lifter needs good hard physical fun. This will help his morale when the gym seems very confining.

Many games can be recommended for lifters. I will list just a few: basketball, soccer, track and field, paddleball, handball, volleyball, gymnastics, swimming, bicycling, ice skating, water and snow skiing, wrestling, hand soccer, diving and the like. The hard contact sports like American football, boxing and lacrosse could produce body contusions which would hinder weightlifting careers; therefore, these sports are not ones to be recommended.

Workout Recovery

As much as possible the waste products built up during training should be removed. In this way the muscles will recover faster and will stand less chance of injury. For this reason hot and cold showers are important. The lifter should get under a hot shower for two or three minutes. The intercellular fluid will then be drawn from the capillaries into the cells because of the high degree of toxicity in the cells. This increase of fluid in the cells will dilute the toxins. Then the lifter should turn the shower to cool or cold (the cooler the better) for 15 seconds.

The cells will constrict (get smaller) and squeeze the excess fluid and toxins out into the intercellular space where it will enter the ciculatory system and be carried off. The lifter should repeat this alternation of hot and cold showers three or four times for best results, ending up with the cool or cold shower.

Another method of removing the waste products is alternating a steam or sauna bath with a swim in a pool or a dip in the snow. If you have never tried this form of recovery, you are in for a pleasant feeling after a workout. There will be much reduced or even no soreness and a real fresh feeling. Taking a hot shower or steam or sauna bath without following it with cool or cold water means excess fluid will get into the cells but will take a long time getting out. It will impinge on nerve fibers because of the stretch of the cells by excess fluid, and there will be increased chance of a muscle cell rupturing. At the same time, the cell is still wallowing in its own filth and not recovering as fast.

Upon waking the morning after a workout, the blood pressure should be taken. If this waking blood pressure is 15% higher than the waking blood pressure of the previous day, then the training for the day should be reduced. When the waking blood pressure returns to normal on a subsequent morning then the lifter can complete his regular workout.

Number of Lifts Per Month Above Certain Key Percentages

The counting of lifts (Olympic lifts and pulls) 90% and above per month has been standard practice. This has been the mainstay for judging proper intensity for many years. We now have the development of counting lifts not only for this percentage but also for the lifts 100% and over. These are not fixed at this time but some fairly accurate figures are available. The body responds to different stimuli for gaining strength. And this new development of counting lifts 100% and over should be viewed with great interest since the Bulgarians pioneered it, and they are the ones who have taken lifters farther toward potential than any other country.

With a good training background, most lifters will be able to fit into their proper category. It must be understood that there are such individual differences as age, years of lifting, high rating despite poor training habits and so on that would make some lifters uncomfortable lifting in the category they qualify for. If such a case occurs, the lifter should be flexible and use the category that seems best for him. He should strive to eventually use the category he properly belongs in. If the individual difference is extreme, then he must operate in the category that seems best. While these are guides which have proven successful, they are flexible.

Preparation Period	Elite	Master	Class I	Class II	Class III	Class IV
90%+	80-100	60-79	40-59	30-39	20-29	10-19
100%	20-30	15-24	12-18	9-13	7-10	5-8
100%+	15-19	12-16	10-13	6-11	5-7	4-6
Contest Period						
90%+	70-85	50-69	30-49	20-29	15-19	10-14
100%	17-25	13-20	10-15	7-11	5-8	4-6
100%+	13-16	10-13	8-12	6-10	4-7	3-5

The 100% and 100%+ lifts are included in the 90%+ counts. The part of the 100% and 100%+ lifts that is the 2 Olympic lifts and the part that is the pulls vary, but the part that is the 2 Olympic lifts does not exceed one third of the counts during the preparation period and one fourth of the counts during the contest period. The pulls therefore comprise at least two thirds of the counts during the preparation period and at least three quarters of the counts during the contest period.

Peaking in Terms of Reps - Bulgaria #5

One of the things discussed at the European Coaches' Conference in Bulgaria was the difficulty in peaking. One of the things associated with this is that when a new lifting season starts, a lifter begins by trying to improve upon his last year's best in the first meet of the season. If he does well, he is proud that he is doing so well so early in the season. And he believes that he will be doing great for the big meets later on. But what invariably happens is that he burns himself out and he does not improve as much as he could have or he even stays the same or regresses.

As was pointed out in the Bulgaria #3 report, the idea of training phases is real, not imaginary. The adrenal glands just will not take the constant whipping to put out. The continual pressure that a lifter puts upon himself to always produce more is keeping his adrenal glands from recuperation. These are the glands that not only get the lifter up for competition but are also responsible for the high performance when he does well. If they do not have a chance to recuperate, the lifter is risking both general health and athletic health (opening himself to such things as pulled or strained muscles).

The first thing to know about peaking is the necessity of slacking off after the regular season with a vacation, and this has already been discussed in the Bulgaria #3 report. Next to know is that in starting a new season, a wise way of peaking would be for the lifter to have as his first cycle goal (if, for example, he is a Class I lifter as described in Bulgaria #3) to total 7-10% less in his first meet than he did for his best the previous season. This means there is less pressure on the lifter physically and mentally, yet it puts him within striking range of his best. The next three peaking cycles the lifter can approach and overtake his best with planned advancements.

The next thing to know about peaking is the necessity of the lifter planning the reps he will use for the season. At the end of this report is a list for lifters in each class; it suggests reps to concentrate on according to which peak cycle the lifter is in. This does not mean that other reps are not done. Rather, these are the reps that most of the sets should be done with. They are broken down into the related exercise groupings described on page 54 of Bulgaria #3. With some exercises, because of their uniqueness, an adjustment up or down of number of reps would have to be made. But the point is that the first peak of the new season does not really zero in on a big total compared to the final peak of the last season because more reps are emphasized at the start. It can be seen that the decrease in reps is gradual and small, but this is very significant. As stated above, the reps outlined are not the only ones done but are those which are being concentrated on at the time. And there is a tremendous difference physically and emotionally from concentrating on triples or doubles rather than singles. Many lifters will say, for example, "I did a double with such and such a weight" or "I did a triple with such and such a weight and, therefore, I should be good for such and such a weight for a single in the contest." When asked how many singles he has done, such a lifter will say none or few, and then in the contest he does not perform his single with the weight he wanted and he wonders why.

When the lifter does doubles or triples, there is less emotional stress than when doing singles. He might think he is getting worked up for a double or triple, but it does not have the same effect on the nervous system and muscular system that a single does. I saw a study by an East German on this. It is something that is very evident but sometimes we overlook it. I am not saying this emotional stress is

bad with singles, just that it is more intense. Singles stimulate progress if:
1) they are not practiced too many times early in the season, 2) they have been pre-
ceded by long periods of higher reps and 3) they fall within a range of 80-95% and
not just a range of 90% and above. Because of the intensity of singles, they can
slow or stop progress if not used wisely.

A lifter should not be lulled into a false sense of security because he is handling good weights for reps. A lifter can get very efficient with reps. There is
the timing, the rhythm and the optimum leverage position one can get into when doing reps that cannot be achieved when doing singles. Thus doubles and triples and
the like are often deceiving when planning a single, unless one has also been doing
a lot of singles. This is not to detract from doing reps and being proud of making
good poundage with reps, because the base is being laid for good singles later if
they too are practiced.

Doing reps and few or no singles can also mean the lifter is over-trained. He
should have been doing singles with weights he was using for doubles and triples.
It is so tempting to do more than one rep with a given weight. For example, an 80%
weight is on the bar and the lifter thinks, "I did one so easy; I'll do more!" However, when he does more, he is not saving his reserves for the next single, and he
starts pacing himself on the first rep so the next rep will go. Therefore, he does
not get an all out explosion for that single. Then when he goes to a contest, he
does not have the backlog of concentration or the correct neuromotor coordination
for doing singles. Many times, such a lifter will be very inconsistent. He almost
paces himself for his three attempts on the platform just as he did with his reps
in training. He might miss his first attempt with a light weight or he might make
only one out of three or two out of three, when he should be making three out of
three.

Doing singles means more than just doing a weight you know you can do (we are
talking about 80% weights). It means total concentration, total coordination for
the one big effort. This is a learned skill, just as the doubles or triples are a
learned skill. Although they are different learned skills, one helps the other up
to a point. When a contest gets near, the lifter needs the most practice on what
he is going to do in the contest. Because reps help build a base for good singles,
a good backlog of reps done early in the season is desirable. As the season goes
on, the lifter should work up to bigger and bigger "peaks" so that when the big contest comes and he is concentrating a lot in his training on singles, then he will
have gotten the most use out of his reps. It works like this: first cycle of peaking - a backlog of reps and then singles for a period; any middle cycle - more
backlog of reps, but not so many as during the first cycle, and then singles for a
period; last cycle - some backlog of reps and then lots of singles.

Singles are certainly important during the contest phase. The lifter should
concentrate on them most when they will do the most good, which is at the end of
the season when the big meets are. Yes, they can be concentrated on early in the
year, but not as much will be gained from them because it is a well known fact that
a backlog of reps is needed to build up good singles. A pretty good peak will be
built up from early concentration on singles, good singles. However, so many times
lifters have wished they had hit their best peaks at the end of the year at the big
contests, instead of earlier in the year at contests which did not mean that much.
When the lifter concentrates more on singles at the beginning of the season, he
peaks early. Not only does a lifter not want to hit a peak early, but also he wants
to get the most benefit possible out of the singles. This comes from doing them
after a backlog of reps.

Strength and power can be gained in two manners: 1) by doing high reps and

2) by doing low reps, with appropriate weights for each. It seems that strength and power are developed when the fast twitch muscle fibers are called into action. This can be done by using heavier weights and lower reps, and it can also be done by using lighter weights and higher reps. When doing high reps, the first reps deplete the glycogen in the slow twitch muscle fibers, and then the fast twitch muscle fibers take over. Using this method of high reps and low weight to build strength and power is very useful to the Olympic lifter because it puts less stress on the joints and offers stimulating change. However, when using this method, the lifter must keep in mind that it is better used on an exercise which does not involve too much coordination (e.g. squats). This is because high reps are fatiguing and coordination is disturbed. Badly coordinated patterns are not a desirable product of gaining strength. High reps and low weight can help the lifter, but he should not use them too often. A proper use of, for example, pre-exhaustion leg work would be once every 7 to 10 days.

On this and the following pages is a chart, according to lifting classification, for suggested reps to concentrate on, depending on what peak cycle the lifter is in. In looking over the suggested reps for the different classes, one thing that becomes apparent is that the lower class lifters do more reps than those in the higher classifications. The thinking behind this is that building a base to get the most out of singles should be like making a pyramid with the most reps done at the lower level and few reps at the top. This gives a long range effect over many years which transcends the season. A backlog of reps for singles is built up during the season's cycles; this is short range. A backlog of reps for singles should also be built up from a lower classification to a higher classification for what we hope will be many seasons; this is long range.

Another thought on this is that as the lifter goes up in classification, he is getting older. This means that he benefits from a lower work load more than when he was younger. This does not mean that gains are not made as one gets older; they certainly are. Some researchers think, for example, that strength can be gained until well into a person's fifties. It just means that an older athlete responds better to less work as he gets older rather than to the same work or more. The Russians thought that this lessening of work ran in 3-5 year periods starting around the mid-twenties.

Cycle of Reps to Concentrate On

Snatch, Clean, Jerk Related Exercises		Leg Related Exercises	Remedial Exercises		
Master & Elite			Leg	Back	Shoulder
Cycle #1 8 wk prep	3	3-4	12-15	8-10	6-8
6 wk contest	2	2-3	8-10	4-6	3-5
Cycle #2 8 wk prep	2-3	3	The above reps for remedial exercises are the same for every class and each cycle of preparation and contest periods.		
6 wk contest	1-2	1-2			
Cycle #3 8 wk prep	2	2			
6 wk contest	1	1-2			
Class I					
Cycle #1 6 wk prep	3	4-5			
5 wk contest	2	3-4			
Cycle #2 6 wk prep	2-3	3-4			
5 wk contest	2	2-3			

Snatch, Clean, Jerk Related Exercises			Leg Related Exercises
Class I (cont.)			
Cycle #3	6 wk prep	2	2-3
	5 wk contest	1-2	1-2
Cycle #4	6 wk prep	2	2
	5 wk contest	1	1-2
Class II			
Cycle #1	5 wk prep	3	5-6
	4 wk contest	2	3-4
Cycle #2	5 wk prep	2-3	4-5
	4 wk contest	2	3
Cycle #3	5 wk prep	2	3-4
	4 wk contest	2	2-3
Cycle #4	5 wk prep	2	2-3
	4 wk contest	1-2	1-2
Class III			
Cycle #1	2-3 wk prep	3	6-7
	4 wk contest	2-3	5-6
Cycle #2	2-3 wk prep	3	5-6
	4 wk contest	2	3-4
Cycle #3	2-3 wk prep	2-3	3-4
	4 wk contest	1-2	2-3
	Vacation		
Cycle #4	2-3 wk prep	3	5-6
	4 wk contest	2	3-4
Cycle #5	2-3 wk prep	2-3	3-4
	4 wk contest	1-2	2-3
Cycle #6	2-3 wk prep	2	2-3
	4 wk contest	1	1-2
Class IV			
Cycle #1	1-2 wk prep	4	7-8
	3 wk contest	3	6-7
Cycle #2	1-2 wk prep	3	6-7
	3 wk contest	2-3	5-6
Cycle #3	1-2 wk prep	3	5-6
	3 wk contest	2	4-5
	Vacation		

Remedial Exercises

Leg	Back	Shoulder
12-15	8-10	6-8
8-10	4-6	3-5

The above reps for remedial exercises are the same for every class and each cycle of preparation and contest periods.

Cycle of Reps to Concentrate On (cont.)

Snatch, Clean, Jerk Related Exercises			Leg Related Exercises	Remedial Exercises		
Class IV (cont.)				Leg	Back	Shoulder
Cycle #5	1-2 wk prep	3	5-6	12-15	8-10	6-8
	3 wk contest	2-3	4-5	8-10	4-6	3-5
Cycle #6	1-2 wk prep	3	4-5			
	3 wk contest	2	3-4			
Cycle #7	1-2 wk prep	2-3	3-4			
	3 wk contest	1-2	2-3			
Cycle #8	1-2 wk prep	2	2-3			
	3 wk contest	1	2			

The above reps for remedial exercises are the same for every class and each cycle of preparation and contest periods.

4

Leg Work - Marseille-Moscow #2

Let me open this report by emphasizing that leg work is not an end in itself. Rather, it is only a means to the end of snatching and clean and jerking more weight.

In the report Bulgaria #3, which had to do with training programs, it was stressed that the theory of training is based on adaptability. An individual's body, based on his inherent characteristics and exposed to what is scientifically and empirically known about training, is brought to adapt to a higher degree of intensity of progressive resistance. The higher degree of intensity one can adapt to, the greater weight he will lift. This report which deals specifically with leg work is no different; it complements the earlier reports. There are some items which will be clarified since this is so specific. Again, not every lifter can fit into a program designed for his level of lifting when he is not used to it. I stressed in earlier reports that it is okay for the lifter to fit into a lower ranking if it feels more comfortable. But from this base point, adaptation to higher levels should take place.

The reader will find a good degree of dependency on high reps (10-20) in doing leg work. This should not create a problem. In Bulgaria #5 it was stated that the fast twitch muscle fibers (which are the power lifting fibers) can be trained by either low or high reps. The other reps recommended are taken from Bulgaria #5 and other past reports.

The theory of specificity is again closely adhered to. This means that as the lifter gets closer to a contest, more things are done like they will be done at the contest. General development because of its broad carry-over value is stressed early in the season and when the contest is far away.

The leg work exercises will be placed into categories. These categories are based on the leg development that is needed for the lifter to make progress in his snatching and clean and jerking. Lifters in the lower classes do exercises in the two most basic and broad categories of this leg development. As they advance in rating, more specific categories are added to hone leg development to its finest for Olympic lifting. Below are listed the categories and their placement into lifting rankings. The number of days per week that leg work is done is taken from Bulgaria #3, namely, Classes III and IV - 2 days per week, Classes I and II - 3 days per week, Master - 4 days per week, and Elite - 5 days per week.

Classes III and IV

    Front Thigh Hip & Upper Thigh

Classes I and II

    Front Thigh Hip & Upper Thigh Speed

Master

    Front Thigh Hip & Upper Thigh Speed Deep Penetrating

Elite

    Front Thigh Hip & Upper Thigh Speed Deep Penetrating Specialized Pull

Next, exercises thought to be among the best will be placed under these categories.

Front Thigh	Hip & Upper Thigh	Speed
1. Front Squat - reps	1. Back Squat, hips in - reps	1. Back Squat - reps
2. Super Killer	2. Back Squat, hips in - reg	2. Front Squat - reps
3. Sissy Squat - reps	3. Back Squat, hips out - reps	3. Back Squat - reg
4. Front Squat - reg	4. Back Squat, hips out - reg	4. Front Squat - reg
5. Hack Squat - reps	5. Back Squat, shoulder straps	5. Throws

Deep Penetrating	Specialized Pull
1. Eccentric	1. Bottom Pull Back Squat, floor
2. Isokinetic	2. Bottom Pull Back Squat, below knee
3. Functional Isometric	3. Top Pull Back Squat, above knee
4. Electro-stimulation	4. Olympic Dead Lift, clean - reps
5. Dead Stops	5. Olympic Dead Lift, clean - reg

These exercises are arranged below based on when the categories under which they fall are practiced within the different classes. The reps are taken from Bulgaria #5 with the exception of high reps, the eccentric reps, isokinetic reps and functional isometric reps. These are dealt with separately in other reports and will be briefly reviewed when a list of the exercises is given later, and peculiarities about them will be discussed. The time - in minutes - allotted to the exercises is under the heading of work and is taken from the Bulgaria #3 report. The intensity at which they are practiced will immediately follow these exercise charts of the six classes.

Class IV

Cycle	Period	Front Thigh Exercise	Reps	Work	Hip & Upper Thigh Exercise	Reps	Work
#1	Prep	Sissy Sq-reps	10-20	12-15	Back Sq, shld strps	7-8	12-15
	Cont	Front Sq-reg	6-7	10	Back Sq, hips in-reg	6-7	10
#2	Prep	Hack Sq-reps	10-20	12-15	Back Sq, hips out-reps	10-20	12-15
	Cont	Front Sq-reg	5-6	10	Back Sq, hips in-reg	5-6	10
#3	Prep	Front Sq-reps	10-20	12-15	Back Sq, hips in-reps	10-20	12-15
	Cont	Front Sq-reg	4-5	10	Back Sq, hips in-reg	4-5	10
#4	Prep	Super Killer	4-5	12-15	Back Sq, hips in-reg	4-5	12-15
	Cont	Front Sq-reg	3-4	10	Back Sq, hips in-reg	3-4	10

Vacation

Cycle	Period	Front Thigh Exercise	Reps	Work	Hip & Upper Thigh Exercise	Reps	Work
#5	Prep	Sissy Sq-reps	10-20	12-15	Back Sq, shld strps	5-6	12-15
	Cont	Front Sq-reg	4-5	10	Back Sq, hips in-reg	4-5	10
#6	Prep	Hack Sq-reps	10-20	12-15	Back Sq, hips out-reps	10-20	12-15
	Cont	Front Sq-reg	3-4	10	Back Sq, hips in-reg	3-4	10
#7	Prep	Front Sq-reps	10-20	12-15	Back Sq, hips in-reps	10-20	12-15
	Cont	Front Sq-reg	2-3	10	Back Sq, hips in-reg	2-3	10
#8	Prep	Super Killer	2-3	12-15	Back Sq, hips in-reg	2-3	12-15
	Cont	Front Sq-reg	2	10	Back Sq, hips in-reg	2	10

Class III

Cycle	Period	Front Thigh Exercise	Reps	Work	Hip & Upper Thigh Exercise	Reps	Work
#1	Prep	Hack Sq-reps	10-20	12-15	Back Sq, hips out-reps	10-20	12-15
	Cont	Front Sq-reg	5-6	12	Back Sq, hips in-reg	5-6	12
#2	Prep	Front Sq-reps	10-20	12-15	Back Sq, hips in-reps	10-20	12-15
	Cont	Front Sq-reg	3-4	12	Back Sq, hips in-reg	3-4	12
#3	Prep	Super Killer	3-4	12-15	Back Sq, hips in-reg	3-4	12-15
	Cont	Front Sq-reg	2-3	12	Back Sq, hips in-reg	2-3	12

Vacation

Cycle	Period	Front Thigh Exercise	Reps	Work	Hip & Upper Thigh Exercise	Reps	Work
#4	Prep	Hack Sq-reps	10-20	12-15	Back Sq, hips out-reps	10-20	12-15
	Cont	Front Sq-reg	3-4	12	Back Sq, hips in-reg	3-4	12
#5	Prep	Front Sq-reps	10-20	12-15	Back Sq, hips in-reps	10-20	12-15
	Cont	Front Sq-reg	2-3	12	Back Sq, hips in-reg	2-3	12
#6	Prep	Super Killer	2-3	12-15	Back Sq, hips in-reg	2-3	12-15
	Cont	Front Sq-reg	1-2	12	Back Sq, hips in-reg	1-2	12

Class II

Cycle	Period	Front Thigh Exercise	Reps	Work	Hips & Upper Thigh Exercise	Reps	Work
#1	Prep	Front Sq-reps	10-20	15	Back Sq, hips out-reps	10-20	15
	Cont	Front Sq-reg	3-4	12-15	Back Sq, hips in-reg	3-4	12-15
#2	Prep	Front Sq-reps	10-20	15	Back Sq, hips out-reps	10-20	15
	Cont	Front Sq-reg	3	12-15	Back Sq, hips in-reg	3	12-15
#3	Prep	Super Killer	3-4	15	Back Sq, hips out-reg	3-4	15
	Cont	Front Sq-reg	2-3	12-15	Back Sq, hips in-reg	2-3	12-15
#4	Prep	Super Killer	2-3	15	Back Sq, hips in-reg	2-3	15
	Cont	Front Sq-reg	1-2	12-15	Back Sq, hips in-reg	1-2	12-15
#5	Prep	Front Sq-reg	2	15	Back Sq, hips in-reg	2	15
	Cont	Front Sq-reg	1-2	12-15	Back Sq, hips in-reg	1-2	12-15

Speed

Cycle	Period	Exercise	Reps	Work
#1	Prep	Back Sq-reps	10-20	15
	Cont	Back Sq-reg	3-4	12-15
#2	Prep	Back Sq-reps	10-20	15
	Cont	Back Sq-reg	3	12-15
#3	Prep	Front Sq-reg	3-4	15
	Cont	Front Sq-reg	2-3	12-15
#4	Prep	Front Sq-reg	2-3	15
	Cont	Front Sq-reg	1-2	12-15
#5	Prep	Front Sq-reg	2	15
	Cont	Throws	1-2	12-15

Class I

Cycle	Period	Front Thigh Exercise	Reps	Work	Hip & Upper Thigh Exercise	Reps	Work
#1	Prep	Front Sq-reps	10–20	20	Back Sq, hips out-reps	10–20	20
	Cont	Front Sq-reg	3–4	15	Back Sq, hips in, reg	3–4	15
#2	Prep	Front Sq-reps	10–20	20	Back Sq, hips out-reg	3–4	20
	Cont	Front Sq-reg	2–3	15	Back Sq, hips in-reg	2–3	15
#3	Prep	Super Killer	2–3	20	Back Sq, hips in-reg	2–3	20
	Cont	Front Sq-reg	1–2	15	Back Sq, hips in-reg	1–2	15
#4	Prep	Front Sq-reg	2	20	Back Sq, hips in-reg	2	20
	Cont	Front Sq-reg	1–2	15	Back Sq, hips in-reg	1–2	15

Speed

Cycle	Period	Exercise	Reps	Work
#1	Prep	Back Sq-reps	10–20	20
	Cont	Back Sq-reg	3–4	15
#2	Prep	Front Sq-reg	3–4	20
	Cont	Front Sq-reg	2–3	15
#3	Prep	Front Sq-reg	2–3	20
	Cont	Front Sq-reg	1–2	15
#4	Prep	Front Sq-reg	2	20
	Cont	Throws	1–2	15

Master

Cycle	Period	Front Thigh Exercise	Reps	Work	Hip & Upper Thigh Exercise	Reps	Work
#1	Prep	Front Sq-reps	10–20	20–25	Back Sq, hips out-reps	10–20	20–25
	Cont	Front Sq-reg	2–3	15–20	Back Sq, hips in-reg	2–3	15–20
#2	Prep	Super Killer	3	20–25	Back Sq, hips in-reg	3	20–25
	Cont	Front Sq-reg	1–2	15–20	Back Sq, hips in-reg	1–2	15–20
#3	Prep	Front Sq-reg	2	20–25	Back Sq, hips in-reg	2	20–25
	Cont	Front Sq-reg	1–2	15–20	Back Sq, hips in-reg	1–2	15–20

Cycle	Period	Speed Exercise	Reps	Work	Deep Penetrating Exercise	Reps	Work
#1	Prep	Back Sq-reps	10–20	20–25	Eccentric	5–6	20–25
	Cont	Back Sq-reg	2–3	15–20	Isokinetic (slow speed)	2–3	15–20
#2	Prep	Front Sq-reg	3	20–25	Functional Isometric 8 stations 6 sec/ea		20–25
	Cont	Front Sq-reg	1–2	15–20	Isokinetic (fast speed)	5–7	15–20
#3	Prep	Front Sq-reg	2	20–25	Eccentric	2–3	20–25
	Cont	Throws	1–2	15–20	Dead Stops	1–2	15–20

Elite

the same as the Master chart with the addition of Specialized Pull

Specialized Pull

Cycle	Period	Exercise	Reps	Work
#1	Prep	Olympic D L, clean-reps	10–20	20–25
	Cont	Olympic D L, clean-reg	2–3	15–20

70

Specialized Pull

Cycle	Period	Exercise	Reps	Work
#2	Prep	Top Pull Back Sq, abv knee	3	20-25
	Cont	Bot Pull Back Sq, bel knee	1-2	15-20
#3	Prep	Bot Pull Back Sq, bel knee	2	20-25
	Cont	Bot Pull Back Sq, floor	1-2	15-20

Intensity

There is a broad but structured guideline for the intensity at which the exercises should be done. Again, it falls under the exercise categories.

Front Thigh   Every 3 workouts a 100% effort should be made for whatever reps are being used. The other 2 workouts should be done in accordance with how the lifter feels but not falling below 75% effort for whatever reps are being used. Once a good warm-up is completed on the 100% day and the 100% is tried, then the lifter should stay as heavy as possible for what time remains in the time slot. A good guideline on the other days is: 1) to work up to a weight that the lifter might have done one or two reps more - one more on a medium day and two more on a light day - when he is doing seven reps or less, and 2) to work up to a weight that the lifter might have done two or three reps more - two more on a medium day and three more on a light day - when he is doing ten reps or more. Once this is reached, then the lifter should stay as heavy as possible using the same guidelines.

Hip & Upper Thigh   Every 5 workouts a 100% effort should be made for whatever reps are being used. The other 4 workouts can be cycled down to 75%. An example would be 75%, 80%, 85%, 92% and 100%, though not necessarily in that order. Once the planned percentage is reached for the day, the lifter should try to stay there for the time that remains in the time slot; he should make an all out effort to do so.

Speed   Every 2 workouts a 90% effort should be made for whatever reps are being used. The other workout an 80-85% effort should be made.

Deep Penetrating   Every 2 workouts an all-out effort should be made for whatever reps are being used. This would mean the following with the different respective deep penetrating exercises:

    Eccentric - 110-140%
    Isokinetic - slowest speed possible but yet movable when using machine; when doing manually each rep takes 6 seconds
    Functional Isometric - all the weight that can be handled, pushed to the top pin and held for 6 seconds
    Dead Stops - all the weight that can be handled from the lifter's respective position with good form

The other workout a sub-effort should be made for whatever reps are being used. This would mean the following with the different respective deep penetrating exercises:

    Eccentric - 95-105%
    Isokinetic - fastest speed possible on machine; when doing manually each rep takes 2 seconds
    Functional Isometric - 85-90% pushed to the top pin and held for 6 seconds
    Dead Stops - 85-90% from the lifter's respective position with good form

There is one other form of deep penetrating exercise called Electro-stimulation. This is done on a machine, and there are several machines put out for this purpose. It is not possible at this time to give a standard intensity for this because the different machines have different electrical modulations. When using any of the machines, the lifter should plan on 2 to 3 training sessions per week.

Specifics of Each Category and Exercise

Most readers of this paper will be familiar with the normal ways of performing the exercises mentioned. I will list here some specific modifications and not all the details of how to do the exercises, which would be repetitious.

One thing should be stressed which is specific to each exercise to be discussed and that is that the lifter should ease into the last two or three inches before the bottom is reached. One of the biggest problems of lifters right now is tendonitis of the patella tendon. Every care should be taken to avoid this because it is so hard to get rid of. Easing into the last two or three inches will mean less weight but more carry-over value to snatching and clean and jerking more weight.

Front Thigh - In all front thigh work the hips should be ahead of the heels, even if this means elevating the heels on a 2-4 inch board. This idea of the hips being ahead of the heels is what is wanted when the lifter is coming up from a clean or even a snatch. Flexibility work should go along with all leg work. Specific flexibility in the Achilles tendon and quadriceps muscles is needed. A gain in flexibility in those places will allow the hips to move ahead of the heels.

Front thigh development is basic in lifting because so much of the intensity of pulling and jerking is felt by the front of the thigh. What often happens when the front thigh development is below par is faulty technique. The practice of front thigh exercises in correct form is essential. Only in this way is there development that is functional to snatching and clean and jerking. Faulty form will result in the exercise not working the front thigh in the manner needed to be of help in the snatch and clean and jerk.

1. Front Squat - reps   Some important points to remember are these: 1) Keep the elbows up and do not let the shoulders round; this has a chance to happen when doing high reps. The rhomboids get stretched and do not get developed, and as a result rounding of the shoulders takes place in the clean and also when jerking. Keep the shoulders up! 2) Ease into the last two or three inches before bottom position is reached. This was stated before, but it should be stated again because when doing reps, the tendency is strong to not ease into those last two or three inches.

2. Front Squat - reg   Remember the points made for exercise #1 because as heavier weights are handled for regular reps, the tendency will also be to round the shoulders and to not ease into the last two or three inches before the bottom. Think speed when doing the regular reps on all weights. Get your neuromuscular system trained to power not strength.

3. Super Killer   This is a front squat done on a 4 inch board with a broom handle or some other long vertical object held by another person behind the lifter between the lifter's heels and a little ahead of them. The lifter's hips are thus well forward. His back should be just about vertical. As he rises he concentrates hard on moving his hips even farther forward. If his hips do come back, they will hit the vertical object. The training partner or whoever is holding the object should not let it move so that the hips must move forward again.

4. Sissy Squats   These have been described in many bodybuilding magazines. The only deviation is to have the feet spaced apart the width they are when coming up from a clean, toes slightly turned out. This exercise is often overlooked by

the Olympic lifter because not much weight can be handled. A tremendous degree of intensity is placed on the front of the thighs. When doing this exercise, keep the knees well forward and do not let the hips even come close to moving back. When more weight is needed, tie it around the waist with a strap or rope.

5. Back Squat Like sissy squats, these have been described over and over in body-building magazines so no further description will be made here. As with the sissy squats, put the feet clean recovery width apart with the toes slightly turned out.

Hip & Upper Thigh - The known role of these muscle areas has increased as the thinking on pulling has evolved. Pulling is now thought of as a hip and thigh lift with the back blending in later on, instead of the back lifting and then the hips and thighs entering in.

Because this type of leg work has general carry-over value to pulling, the hips when doing this work are sometimes permitted to go back since they are worked more this way, as is the upper thigh. But because of specificity, at various times the hips are also not allowed to go back because they do not go back when pulling. In other words, general overload is wanted at certain times and then, to get as much carry-over value as possible, specific overload is wanted at other times. Take a stance as close to a clean recovery stance as possible when doing the exercises, with the toes slightly pointed out.

1. Back Squat, hips in - reps Have the bar placed high on the traps and not low on the shoulders. This will encourage a more upright back position and thus the hips will be in more. In many instances the hips will not be able to be ahead of the heels but should be as far forward as possible even if a 2-4 inch board is needed. Ease into the last two or three inches before bottom. Thrusting the elbows forward when coming up will also help keep a more upright position and keep the hips in.

2. Back Squat, hips in - reg Remember the same points covered in exercise #1.

3. Back Squat, hips out - reps The bar can rest low on the shoulders for this. This will encourage the hips to be back. Much more weight can be handled, as much as or more than 100 pounds, than with the hips in. More strain will be on the lower back since the back tilts forward more. Do not use more weight than the lower back will stand. If pain develops, use less weight. Previous work should have included lower back work to prepare for such an exercise.

4. Back Squat, hips out - reg Remember the same points covered in exercise #3.

5. Back Squat, shoulder straps This exercise is used with a piece of equipment like the Magic Circle, which is described in Iron Man magazine. There are two wide straps that go over the lifter's shoulders and with hooks or snaps attach to a barbell or some such supportive apparatus onto which weights can be loaded. It is used mainly with beginners to give them a dispersed feeling of weight on their shoulders instead of the concentrated one that a barbell gives. But it can also be used with more advanced lifters. This equipment distributes the weight over a broader base and puts less strain on the shoulders. Good squatting technique, either with the hips in or out, is thought to be achieved quicker with this exercise. For more detailed use of this equipment, I refer the reader to the article on page 111, Magic Circle. (Please note that I do not sell this equipment for Iron Man or in any way get financial remuneration from the sale of this piece of equipment.)

Speed - Speed exercises cannot be emphasized enough. There are many lifters with strong legs. That means they can come up with heavy weights when squatting. But there are fewer lifters who can come up with a little less weight when squatting but with great speed. Pulling is a fast motion, and coming up from a clean should be a fast motion. These movements take leg <u>power</u>, and that means speed. You can train a muscle to move fast. Neurologically, if you think speed your muscles will contract faster. Speed is specific. If you squat with heavier and heavier weights while not paying attention to speed, you will get stronger with heavier and heavier weights. But your legs will not get more power for the athletic speed you need to clean or snatch a heavy weight. I am not discounting squatting with heavy weights and grinding out the reps. Apparently, what this does is activate deep muscle fibers. However, after they are activated, they must be trained for speed if the strength developed is to be converted into the power needed for the lifting of heavy weights in the snatch and clean and jerk.

When doing speed exercises, the lifter should have someone help him by using a stop watch. As the lifter starts to rise from the low position, the watch is started. As his knees straighten at the top, the watch is stopped. Then the watch is started again when he has returned to the bottom and starts up once more. Sporting goods stores sell stop watches which accumulate time. Again, ease in at the bottom! Do not crash or even slow down at the bottom; ease in.

These speed exercises, besides building power for snatching and clean and jerking, are fun. It is a real challenge to try to beat your previous time. It is a new incentive. These exercises also take the strain off the lower back since a lighter weight is handled. The back feels more alive and fresh. In all speed squats the hips should be in. Nothing new need be said about any but one of the exercises since a referral back to similar exercises points out what should be paid attention to.

1. Throws   The bar is at the shoulders and the lifter goes down as he would be doing for a normal front squat. After easing in at the bottom, he then accelerates as fast as possible with sufficient power to throw the bar off his shoulders high enough so that he can catch the bar on his traps. If more than one rep is called for, he then goes into a normal back squat and then accelerates as fast as possible with sufficient power to throw the bar off his traps high enough that he can catch the bar on his shoulders. It may seem at first that not enough weight can be used to truly call this a leg building exercise, but remember that power is using strength quickly enough to be able to pull a weight to a sufficient height or to come up from a clean easily; as long as there is progressive resistance (more and more weight as the body adapts) then power will be developed. If this exercise is done correctly, especially with reps, the thighs really feel worked. It will take a few times to get the timing down to be able to catch the weight in the right spot and without any jarring. Give in with the legs a little as the bar is coming down, and this will cushion the catch.

<u>Deep Penetrating</u> - These are the exercises that have been shown by physiological studies to activate more muscle fibers than do normal kinds of progressive resistance. Many times muscle fibers would never have been activated if it were not for these exercises. Some physiologists believe they are so deeply penetrating because the natural defense mechanism of the body, which prevents a person from contracting a muscle so hard as to hurt himself, is partially bypassed. It is not entirely bypassed since there seems to be enough natural defense in operation to keep from getting hurt, because the injury rate from these exercises is no greater than from normal exercises.

1. Eccentric   This is basically lowering the weight under control. In the squatting exercises suggested for legs, the lifter bends his knees and slowly gives

in to the weight so that after 6 seconds he has bent his knees enough to be in a full squat position. The incentive is to use more and more weight in correct form for 6 seconds. If the lowering is faster than 6 seconds, then too much weight is being used. Naturally, spotters are needed to help the lifter up from this full squat position so that another rep can be done.

There is an Eccentric Machine sold by Bob Michaels, World Fitness Center, Inc. at 2013 Pioneer Boulevard in Lincoln, Nebraska. This machine is run by a motor. Two ropes are attached to the bar and when the motor is on, it pulls the bar down. The lifter is under the bar and tries to slow down the bar. Someone can time how long it takes for the motor to pull the bar down; the incentive is for the lifter to increase this time. The longer the time, the stronger the lifter is becoming because he is resisting the motor longer. (Please note that I do not work for this company and get no financial remuneration from the sale of this machine.)

2. Isokinetic   This is constant resistance throughout the whole movement. Therefore, the lifter works his strong areas of movement in addition to his weak ones. In normal exercises with a barbell, usually only the weak areas are worked hard, because when they are, they give out and the exercise cannot be continued; this leaves the strong areas not given as much work.

There is a company called Mini-Gym at Box 266 in Independence, Missouri, which sells an isokinetic ham-quad unit. The unit has multiple speeds. The slow speeds work the deepest muscle fibers, and the faster speeds train the fibers to be more powerful. As stated during the section on intensity, both of the speeds need to be used. (Again, I do not sell machines for this company.) A leg press unit can also be bought to complement the ham-quad unit.

The quadriceps can also be worked isokinetically by manual resistance. A partner puts his hands on the lifter's foot and pushes down evenly as the lifter tries to straighten his knee. If using a training partner for manual resistance, a lifter can assume various positions in which he can straighten or flex his knees, extend his hips or abduct his thighs. Please refer to other parts of this report for intensity and work suggested.

Isokinetic movement isolates muscles that are normally used in their entirety when the lifter is doing some sort of pull or squat. Therefore, whether the isokinetics are done manually or with a machine, it is advisable when doing them to work the quads, the thigh biceps, the hips and possibly the outsides of the thighs.

3. Functional Isometric   With the bar between two pins one hole apart on each side, the bar is pushed up from the lower pin and held against the upper pin for 6 seconds. The movement of the squat should be divided into 8 equal distances apart and one rep per distance should be done. The incentive on a maximum day is to hold heavier and heavier weights against the top pin for 6 seconds. In all distances, keep the hips in. Use the back squat.

4. Electro-stimulation   As stated before, these machines are used 2 to 3 times a week, and the major muscle groups of the hips and thighs are worked. It seems that each machine is modulated a little differently from the others. Some areas which have used this with success are the Pennsylvania, Maryland and Los Angeles areas. For further information, I suggest the reader contact: Dick Smith, c/o York Barbell Company, Box 1707, York, Pennsylvania 17405; Dr. John Ziegler, 17812 Princess Ann Drive, Olney, Maryland 20832; Bob Hise, Sr., Box 54204, Los Angeles, California 90055, or myself at 302 Chula Vista, Santa Fe, N.M. 87501.

5. Dead Stops   With the bar resting on the pins in a power rack and on the traps, and the lifter one to two inches from dead bottom, he drives up fast to complete extension. After finishing the reps at that position, he puts the bar on pins set at a height so that the thigh bone is right above parallel; he drives up fast for the required reps. Then he sets the bar on pins so that the body is 4-6 inches lower than full height; he drives up for the required reps. Thus there are three positions. In all positions keep the hips in, and use the back squat.

Specialized Pull - These leg exercises are very specific in working the legs along the lines they will be used when pulling. They add a lot to the leg program by using the leg power already gained and zeroing in on exactly what is going to be done in competition. Because they are specific and their value lies in their specificity, adherence to correct execution of them is of great importance.

1. Bottom Pull Back Squat, floor   With the bar on his traps the lifter assumes the position he would be in if he was going to pull the bar from the floor. From here he nearly straightens, then rebends and straightens his knees as if he were doing the double knee bend. The hard part here will be to keep the hips from shooting out back and to have the shoulders go forward enough when the bar - if there were a bar being pulled - passes the knees. The lifter accelerates the movement as height is gained. After the rebending when the hips go down and forward, there is a marked increase in leverage and great acceleration can take place. After the knees straighten, the lifter goes up on his toes and remains there for 3 seconds. Remaining on the toes for 3 seconds means that the forces to extension add upward and not forward or backward.

2. Bottom Pull Back Squat, below knee   With the bar on his traps the lifter assumes the position he would be in if he were going to pull the bar from 2-3 inches below the knee. From here he nearly straightens the knee, then rebends and straightens his knees, as described in exercise #1. Everything else is done like exercise #1.

3. Top Pull Back Squat, above knee   With the bar on his traps the lifter assumes the position he would be in if he were going to pull the bar from 2-3 inches above his knees. From here he bends his knees (as in the rebend in exercises #1 and #2), then straightens them and goes up on his toes as in exercise #1.

4. Olympic Dead Lift, clean - reps   This should be done exactly like the double knee bend and with straps. When done this way, it gives the thighs a tremendous workout. When form is broken, then the back is worked which is not wanted. There is no shrug done here. The weight is lowered after the knees straighten, and another rep is started.

5. Olympic Dead Lift, clean - reg   This is no different from the previous exercise. Since more weight is used, and a lot of weight can be used, strict adherence to good form is a must.

5

Peaking Intensities - Marseille-Moscow #3

Within the contest phase, discussed at length in Bulgaria #3, there are peaking intensities. These are thought to be very critical. With proper previous training in the preparation phase and at the beginning of the contest phase the lifter should be ready to bring everything to bear to get the most out of his body at that particular time of the year by following proper peaking intensities. This is done quite successfully in Europe because they have had a lot of experience with trying out different peaking intensities two to three weeks before a contest. In putting forth some of the suggested peaking intensities, certain aspects need explanation.

Different classes react differently to different peaking intensities. In the lighter classes a higher peaking intensity can be tried closer to the contest. In the heavier classes more time to recuperate from a higher peaking intensity is needed. Also, it is harder for a heavier class lifter to develop speed. By using lighter weights as the contest approaches he can concentrate and train more on speed. He needs more speed work than does the lighter class lifter.

The classes are grouped according to how they seem to have reacted in the past to different peaking intensities. For this reason the 114-132 pound classes are grouped together, the 148 and 165 pound classes are grouped together, the 181-242 pound classes are grouped together, and the super-heavyweights are by themselves. Naturally, there are deviations from this. When guidelines are made such as these, they are done so because of a general over-all trend that is significant, knowing full well that a small proportion of lifters will have to be treated individually.

In the charts of suggested peaking intensities are listed percentages. These percentages mean various things depending on what lifts or work they are referring to. In the snatch and snatch pull it means percentage of what the lifter wants to snatch at the coming contest. Similarly, in the clean and jerk and the clean pull it means percentage of what the lifter wants to clean at the coming contest. Leg work percentages refer to percentage of the lifter's best for those reps being done. In jerk work the percentages vary since the jerk work is split up into three movements. These are: 1) Heavy Partial Movements (e.g. jerk drives, recoveries) - for these it is the percentage of what the lifter wants to jerk at the next contest, 2) Simulated Jerk Movements (e.g. push up and out, push jerk) - for these it is the percentage of those reps being followed at the time, and 3) Technique Movements (e.g. jerk off the rack, front squat and jerk) - for these it is the percentage of what the lifter wants to jerk at the next contest.

The suggested reps to be used for the peaking intensities should be found in the Bulgaria #5 and Marseille-Moscow #2 reports, remembering that these are not the only reps that are done but are the main reps being used during the cycle that the lifter is in.

Once the peaking intensities in any given exercise are worked up to, the rest of the time allocated to that exercise should be used. If weights are being used which are 80% or above, then the lifter should not drop down to less than 80%. If weights are used which are below 80% (which they will be with only 1-3 days before competition), then the lifter should stay at the peaking intensity suggested.

Within the suggested peaking intensities is a deviation of 2% up or down. This deviation is based on the cardiovascular fitness of the lifter. If the lifter is in good cardiovascular shape, then he might be able to lift with a 2% higher peaking

intensity in many of the exercises. If he is not in good cardiovascular shape, then
he might have to lift with a 2% lower peaking intensity in many of the exercises.

The question then becomes, what is good cardiovascular shape or fitness? There
are all sorts of elaborate ways of finding this out, but a good practical test is
the Harvard Step Test. It is easy to take; a person can do it by himself with a
small chair or bench and a clock with a second hand. This test can be obtained by
writing to the American Association for Health, Physical Education and Recreation,
1201 16th Street NW, Washington, D.C. 20036.

One of the big frontiers in Olympic Weightlifting is peaking correctly for a
contest. Even the wisest have trouble getting the most out of their bodies consistently. The following charts are guidelines which should help lifters peak correctly
and lift better in their contests.

Peaking Intensity Percentage Guidelines

114-132 Weight Classes

Days Before Contest	Snatch	C&J	Sn Pull	Cl Pull	Leg	Heavy Partial Movements	Sim. Jerk Movements	Technique Movements
10-12	100+	100+	110	105	100+	115	100+	100+
8-9	97	95	107	105	100+	110	95	95
6-7	95	90	102	100	90	105	90	90
4-5	90	85	100	95	85	100	85	85
3	85	80	95	90	80	-	-	-
2	80	75	90	85	75	-	-	-
1	70	65	-	-	-	-	-	-

148 & 165 Weight Classes

Days Before Contest	Snatch	C&J	Sn Pull	Cl Pull	Leg	Heavy Partial Movements	Sim. Jerk Movements	Technique Movements
13-14	100+	100+	110	107	100+	117	100+	100+
11-12	97	95	107	105	100+	112	95	95
9-10	97	95	107	102	97	107	92	95
7-8	95	90	105	100	95	102	90	90
5-6	92	87	100	97	90	97	87	87
4	87	82	97	92	82	92	82	82
3	82	77	92	87	77	-	-	-
2	77	72	87	82	72	-	-	-
1	70	65	-	-	-	-	-	-

181-242 Weight Classes

Days Before Contest	Snatch	C&J	Sn Pull	Cl Pull	Leg	Heavy Partial Movements	Sim. Jerk Movements	Technique Movements
15-17	100+	100+	115	110	100+	120	100+	100+
12-14	97	95	110	105	100+	112	95	95
9-11	95	90	105	100	95	105	90	90
6-8	92	87	100	95	90	100	85	87
4-5	87	85	95	90	85	90	80	85
3	80	75	90	85	77	-	-	-
2	75	70	85	80	72	-	-	-
1	67	62	-	-	-	-	-	-

Super-Heavy Weight Class

Days Before Contest	Snatch	C&J	Sn Pull	Cl Pull	Leg	Heavy Partial Movements	Sim. Jerk Movements	Technique Movements
18-20	100+	100+	117	112	100+	125	100+	100+
15-17	97	95	112	107	100+	117	97	95
12-14	95	92	107	102	97	110	95	92
10-11	92	90	105	100	92	102	90	90
8-9	90	85	102	100	90	95	85	85
6-7	85	82	97	95	87	87	80	82

Super-Heavy Weight Class (cont.)

Days Before Contest	Snatch	C&J	Sn Pull	Cl Pull	Leg	Heavy Partial Movements	Sim. Jerk Movements	Technique Movements
4-5	82	80	92	90	82	-	-	-
3	77	75	87	82	75	-	-	-
2	72	67	82	77	70	-	-	-
1	65	60	-	-	-	-	-	-

Cycle Examples

Cycle #1 Class I Program

Day	Exercise	Reps – Prep	Reps – Contest
1	Snatch, floor	3	2
	Power Snatch	3	2
	Jerk Off Rack	3	2
	Back Squats	5	3
	Hypers	8-10	4-6
2	Clean and Jerk	1cl 1j 1cl	2cl 1j
	Snatch off boxes, below knee	3	2
	Power Clean	3	2
	Push Jerk	3	2
	Leg Extension, Leg Curl	12-15	8-10
3	Front Squat and Jerk	1sq 1j 1sq 1j	1sq 1j
	On Toes, Split and Recover	3	2
	Ascending Snatch Pull	3	2
	Speed Squat	5	3
	Press, behind neck	6-8	3-5
	Hypers	8-10	4-6
4	Clean and Jerk	1cl 2j	1cl 1j
	Snatch off boxes, right below mid-thigh	3	2
	Press, out and up	3	2
	Ascending Clean Pull	3	2
	Leg Extension, Leg Curl	12-15	8-10
5	Clean, floor	3	2
	Super Killer Squat, front	5	3
	Jerk Drive	3	2
	High Pull Snatch	3	2
	High Pull Clean	3	2
	Press, behind neck	6-8	3-5

One Month Example
Placement of 90%+ Lifts

Day	Lifts	Day	Lifts
1	1	11	4
2	2	12	2
3	1	13	2
4	3	14	2
5	4	15	1
6	2	16	2
7	3	17	2
8	3	18	3
9	2	19	2
10	1	20	3

Cycle #2 Class I Program

Day	Exercise	Reps - Prep	Reps - Contest
1	Snatch, 1 floor, the rest hang	2-3	2
	Stiff Knee Power Snatch, 1 floor the rest hang	2-3	2
	Jerk Balance	2-3	2
	Back Squat, hips out	3-4	2-3, hips in
	Hypers	8-10	4-6
2	Clean and Jerk	1cl 2j	1cl 2j
	Snatch off boxes, right below mid-thigh	2-3	2
	Stiff Knee Power Clean	2-3	2
	Push Jerk	2-3	2
	Leg Extension, Leg Curl	12-15	8-10
3	Front Squat and Jerk	1sq 2j	1sq 2j
	On Toes, Split and Recovery	2-3	2
	Ascending Snatch Pulls	2-3	2
	Speed Squat	3-4	2-3
	Stiff Knee Power Snatch to Forehead and Press Out	6-8	3-5
	Hypers	8-10	4-6
4	Clean and Jerk	1cl 2j	1cl 1j
	Snatch, 1 floor, the rest hang	2-3	2
	Press, out and up	2-3	2
	Ascending Clean Pulls	2-3	2
	Leg Extension, Leg Curl	12-15	8-10
5	Clean, 1 floor, the rest hang	2-3	2
	Front Squat	10-20	2-3
	Jerk Drive	2-3	2
	Power Clean, snatch grip	3	2
	High Pull Clean	2-3	2
	Stiff Knee Power Snatch to Forehead and Press Out	6-8	3-5

Placement of 90%+ lifts can be done as in Cycle #1.

Daily Record Sheet Example

Exercises	Date & Day_____					Date & Day_____				
Snatch Related	Weight	Reps	Sets	Work	# 90% Lifts	Weight	Reps	Sets	Work	# 90% Lifts
Clean Related										
Jerk Related										
Leg Work										
Miscellaneous										
	Weight	Reps	Sets	Work	# 90% Lifts	Weight	Reps	Sets	Work	# 90% Lifts
TOTAL										

K Value Revisited

Earlier I wrote an article entitled "Wanted - K Values of American Lifters". In the article I tried to explain what the K value is and what its merits are, and I asked for American lifters to calculate their K values and send them to me. Much has happened since then which I would like to relate.

I will begin by saying that during my trips to Europe and Mexico City this past summer (1974), my talks with coaches from Germany, France, Spain, England, Mexico and Cuba emphasized again the great importance of the K value. These coaches agree that after style is developed or even as style is being developed, the best way to increase strength is to train at the correct intensity. This is the way the body responds. It is not blasted into strength, and neither is it loafed into strength. The K value gives the relationship of the amount of intensity to what the lifter can realistically expect to total in the two Olympic lifts. Let us look at what is involved.

$K = \frac{Ia \times 100}{Total}$ is the formula. Ia is the intensity. This is calculated by adding up all the poundage and dividing by all the reps. This is the average amount of weight lifted every time a weight is lifted; it is the average intensity the lifter is training at. It is this average intensity that is either going to stimulate the body to get stronger or not get stronger. And there is a relationship between this average intensity and what one can realistically expect to do in the next competition. This relationship is called the K value.

You can see that if your average intensity goes up and your total is the same, then a higher K value results. If the average intensity goes down and your total is the same, then the K value goes down. These and other forms of deviations result because something over something else is a relationship just as 10 over 2 is 5 and 8 over 2 is 4.

In a practical weightlifting example, let us say that a lifter wants to total 700 at the next contest (maybe by way of 300-400). Let's say he adds up all his poundage and it totals 25,500 pounds, and he adds up all his reps and they add up to 100. Dividing 25,500 by 100 he comes up with an average intensity of 255. To find the K value he plugs in the numbers to the K value formula and this is $K = \frac{255 \times 100}{700}$. Working this out results in a K value of 36.43. Now let us say that during another period of training months later, the same lifter still wants to make a realistic 700 total. He adds up all his tonnage and it comes to 30,000 pounds. He adds up all his reps and they come to 125. Dividing 30,000 by 125 gives an average intensity of 240. During this period his average intensity was lowered 15 pounds from the earlier 255 pounds. Again plugging into the equation of K = Ia x 100 divided by Total, we have K = 240 x 100 divided by 700 and the result is 34.3. Did the lifter make more progress when his K value was 36.43 or when it was 34.3? In other words, what we are saying is did he make more progress when he was lifting with more average intensity in comparison to what he could realistically do, or did he make more progress when he was lifting with less average intensity in comparison to what he could realistically do? Here lies the value of the K. If the lifter can establish a trend for a certain K value, then he can adjust his workouts to always have that K value.

Continuing with the same example of this hypothetical lifter, let us say he does make the 700 total with a K value of 36.43. Next contest he thinks he can make 730. To keep the same K value he must readjust his average intensity (Ia). To do so he would plug in the known values to the equation K = Ia x 100 divided by Total, namely 36.43 = Ia x 100 divided by 730, and the result is Ia = 266 pounds. This means he must now adjust his reps and poundages so that his average intensity comes out to be 266 pounds. This will give him the same relationship of intensity lifted in workouts to what he can realistically hope to do in a contest (730) as he had when he wanted to realistically total 700. This adjustment is an easy thing to do. It takes about 30 minutes to figure out. With a pocket calculator it takes less.

I cannot stress enough the importance of planning around the K value. It is a basic tool. Many people do not use it because it seems like too much work, but whatever time you spend on it is justified, and it really does not require an excessive amount of time. At a National Junior Olympic Training Camp some of the younger boys 11 and 12 years old were doing such planning in a matter of minutes once they understood it and tried it out. It is not that much work and it is one of the two most important guides (the other being counting reps over 90% of the two Olympic lifts and related lifts, e.g. pulls) in figuring how heavy one should lift in training. Intensity is the key. Once suitable tonnage is reached, progress will be made only if the intensity is increased; the amount to increase can best be known through the K value.

Now that we have come this far, let me give some other guides for using the K value. First, in counting the amount of pounds and reps for figuring the intensity, you should count all exercises with the exception of exercises which involve ridiculously small weights as in sit-ups, wrist curls and the like.

Second, in counting the amount of pounds for figuring the intensity, you should count only those weights and reps that figure out to be 60% or more of what you realistically want to do the next contest. This means basing pulls on this also. The pulls are figured as based on what you want to snatch or clean, not what your best snatch or clean pull is. It is 60% of your expected snatch and 60% of your expected clean.

Third, in figuring your total, be realistic. A good rule of thumb is that after the lifting season is over, take your best total and subtract 7 to 10 percent of it for your first goal of the coming season. Then build from there. This would be the first part of a cycling season. This subtraction gives you many things, one being a psychological rest. You do not want to burn out early in the season. This backing off of your best performance is done so often in other sports. It also gives you a physical rest. This is so important; the body needs this "active" physical rest. It just does not respond to driving it to new heights all year.

Fourth, figure the K value normally on a monthly basis. If you are preparing for a contest for which you are peaking and not treating as just another workout, figure it on a weekly basis from week 6 through week 2 before the contest. Usually there is a 2% increase from week 6 through week 2 in final peaking.

We have had good response to our call for K values of American lifters. It turns out that the best progress in the United States is being made on K values of between 32% and 38%. Western European, Mexican and Cuban coaches all told me that they have observed the best progress being made by Eastern European countries on K values of 40%. The higher value could be from the lifters there being in better shape so that they can recover from a higher intensity workout.

This brings me to a last but important point. Early in your lifting year you must get in shape. Run dashes, bicycle, swim, high jump, broad jump, play soccer, play volleyball or play basketball on a regular basis. This being in shape early in the lifting year is one of the important things that will enable you to train at an optimum K value as the year progresses. You want to recover from those intensity workouts, and this means getting in shape early in the year. Then a little bit of such conditioning later in the year will suffice to keep that good condition. Get your heart strength and blood vessel strength at a time when there is not that pressure to lift top poundages, and you will see how it pays off later in the year.

9

Leg Work for the Olympic Lifter

In this article I will discuss exercises that pertain to specific work on the legs. Such exercises fit into the cycling system. You do not count the number of reps over 90% when doing leg exercises, but you do figure the intensity of leg work in the cycling when you are figuring the K value.

What I am about to explain is relatively new in the United States, but it is not new overseas; it has long been practiced by the Europeans. They believe in working around the spine and knees so that they will remain fresh and not get hurt. An example in the United States is the work of Bob Hise with Roger Quinn in performing manual isokinetic exercises for the legs. Both men have indicated in conversations with me that Roger's leg strength is better than before and his knees feel much better.

Doing squats, squats and more squats in the same manner is really debilitating to the spine and knees. After all the pulls and low positions a lifter hits, it is a wonder his spine and knees can take any squats at all. Certainly after a few years something will probably give. Why not vary the routine? By varying, I do not mean alternating light, medium and heavy squats, although this is better variation than none at all. Instead, I mean doing something like speed squats, leg work that isolates the muscles of the knees and hips without straining the knees and spine, and such work as pre-exhaustion leg work which accomplishes the same thing.

For example, let us say you are going to work legs four times a week. On day number one you might do your regular squats. You may be doing front or back squats for 3's or 5's, but let us assume that you will get in 4 weeks of day-one squatting during a month. One week you should work up to 70% of your best for the amount of reps you are doing. During week number two, do 80%. During week number three do 90%. Then during week number four try for a record.

Continuing the example, on day number two you might do speed squats. You should take 80% of your best for the number of reps you are doing and see how fast you can do these. The Russians were doing a form of these many years ago. For this you need someone to time you. Because you are only competing against yourself, your down rhythm should be kept constant so that only your up or rising rhythm is the one that goes faster. If you increase dropping speed you will bang into the bottom. Do seven sets in the following manner. Warm up for three sets and then on the fourth, fifth and sixth sets have yourself timed, using 80% of your best for the number of reps you are doing at the time. A seventh set can be added using a lighter weight and doing it without being timed, just a cooling down set. This really adds power to your legs, and that is what lifters want. They should not be trying to see how much they can front squat with. They need to be able to use their hips, legs and lower back with explosiveness. These speed squats give that explosion, that power.

On day number three you can work around the knees with such leg and hip exercises as leg presses on a machine, sissy squats (for the front of the thighs which really play an important role in rising out of a heavy clean or dipping with the rear end in when jerking), leg extensions and even leg curls. These can be done on conventional machinery or on isokinetic machinery, or they can be done using isokinetics manually like Bob Hise does with Roger Quinn. With the exception of doing these using isokinetics manually and on isokinetic machines for which 3 to 5 reps for one to two sets is sufficient, usually four sets of 12 reps is recommended when blending into the total four days of leg work.

On day four the pre-exhaustion leg work can be done. In a study of the front squat other people have found, as I myself did, that only 30% of the strength in the front squat comes from the quads. The rest comes mainly from the lower back and upper hip. So imagine what this percentage would be if one did back squats during which even more weight is borne by the spine. Therefore, what tires first is the lower back, and the legs do not really get worked. The theory of pre-exhaustion leg work is that the lifter completely exhausts the quads and then squats. This can be done by leg extensions, a set of leg presses and then squatting. Again, with the exception of manual and machine isokinetic work during which lower reps will exhaust the quads sooner, a set of 8 to 12 reps is done. Then choose a weight that is about 60% of your best for 5 reps in the squat and do as many reps as you can. Once 10-15 reps is reached, increase the weight for the squat.

Does this sound strange? Really it is not. As I said, foreign lifters have been doing variations of this for years. Some lifters may think that in some cases the reps are too high, but some of our best lifters have said they have made their best leg gains with high reps. The above leg routine is only one of many variations. My main concern is that some such variation be used as a change from the constant blasting of the spine and knees which leaves them dead or hurting after a few years. For an Olympic lifter there are better ways of training the legs than to continue doing squats workout after workout. With these better ways comes better progress and a spine that is alive and has whip, and knees that have spring instead of pain.

Eccentric Contraction

Eccentric contraction is lowering the weight under control. There are two main reasons for using it. One is that it involves more muscle fibers than any other form of progressive resistance. The other is that it is a possible teaching aid for developing style, used as an extra emphasis.

This type of contraction can be used with both conventional weights and the Power Master Eccentric Machine. The latter can be obtained through Bob Michaels at the World Fitness Center, Inc., 2013 Pioneer Boulevard in Lincoln, Nebraska. With conventional weights it can be used for whole movements and partial movements. You do four to six sets of 1 to 6 reps, and you do it once every 7 to 10 days. Every whole rep lasts 6 seconds; partial reps last 4 seconds. With the Eccentric Machine it can also be used for whole movements and partial movements. You do two to three sets of 1 to 3 reps, and you do it once every 7 to 10 days. The incentive here is to time the movements with a stop watch (both whole and partial movements); the machine will slow down with greater resistance.

On Using Water and Static Flexibility Exercises
for Short and Long Term Flexibility Gains

In Bulgaria #3 report (Training Methods) I discussed static flexibility exercises for immediate and long term flexibility gains, and I discussed the use of water for recuperation after a workout. I would now like to discuss the role both play when used together in immediate and long term flexibility gains.

In the last decade the idea of hot moist heat penetrating deeply was justifiably challenged. In the body circulatory system there are arterial shunts which can move blood to different areas. It seems that hot moist heat opens up the arterial shunts to the skin and much of the blood then passes into and through the muscles into the skin; this does not greatly help the athlete. Due to this discovery, taking hot showers before working out was no longer advocated for the purpose of helping muscles become more flexible because of more warm blood to them. While the athlete felt better when he took a hot shower because this was a nice sensation to the skin receptors, it did not do a lot to increase the blood flow to his muscles. In fact it gave him a false sense of security because while he felt loose, it was just the good feeling in his skin and not because his muscles were warm and could thus move a greater range.

With the discrediting of hot showers, warm showers were then tried (water from 90°-100° F.). Tests revealed that with a warm shower there is indeed an increase in blood flow to the muscles which stays there for most part and is not shunted off to the skin. It was also found that after a warm shower the muscles can be stretched more than if no heat were applied or if hot heat were applied. In addition, it was found that after a warm shower temporary cartilage cells form around the joints and give added protection for a stressful competition or workout.

Another finding is the importance of doing static flexibility exercises immediately after the warm shower, at which time such exercises can be of the greatest benefit to an athlete. These are exercises which, either through an athlete's own pressure or with the aid of a training partner, push a given body part to the end point of flexibility, slowly, and then a little bit beyond where it is held for 10 seconds, relaxed for 1 or 2 seconds, and then returned to beyond the end point of flexibility for another 10 seconds. This is repeated 5 or 6 times. This should be done for ankles, knees, hips, groins, back, shoulders and wrists. Static flexibility allows a given muscle to be stretched farther than it can be stretched using other forms of stretching exercises. (This is partly because the opposing muscle is not called into play, which would limit the length of stretch.) Furthermore, the most stretch is obtained when such exercises follow the warm shower.

All this was taken from the physical therapy profession and applied to weightlifting as well as to other sports. What happens is that by using this procedure, more immediate flexibility is gained for warming-up and more long term flexibility is gained, if practiced regularly, than any gain from previous forms of flexibility work practiced. It is really a sight to see some of these warm-ups take place. Your first impression might be that you do not know what the athletes are trying to accomplish except that they are very clean from taking showers and they seem to be into some type of Yoga! But, of course, there is much more to it, as you now understand from reading this article. There are definite short and long term flexibility gains to be had by preceding a workout or competition with a warm, not hot, shower and following the shower with static flexibility exercises.

SECTION IV

THE CONTEST AND BEFORE

1

Backstage

Starting Poundage

This depends on how you are moving and your reflexes. You should not be locked in mentally by a certain weight. Try to put pressure on the other guy by forcing him to take better than his best. Do not forget that World Record poundages which you read about have been exceeded in the gym, so doing it on the platform is no big deal. Remember that your goal is to lift the best you can that day with what you have. If the peak is right, then you will set new personal bests; if it is not, then you will still have positive success by making many attempts. Many attempts made means a base for record poundages that meet or in later meets.

Warm-ups

Stretch for about 15-20 minutes, preferably manual stretching and with warm water applied first to ankle and wrist joints. Take 3-4 minutes between sets. Work up to 20-35 pounds under your starting attempt (less if more confidence is needed). At most do 2 reps with light weights, then singles with heavy weights. The last warm-up should be about 5 minutes before your first attempt. In a contest where there is a long wait, every 3-5 minutes do a lift with 80-85%. This lift need not be complete. For example, snatch the weight but do not come up; dump it. Clean the weight but do not come up; dump it. Five or six sets of warm-ups after a general warm-up is good for the snatch, four or five sets for the clean and jerk.

Do not sit for more than $3\frac{1}{2}$ minutes; get up and move around. Keep the joints free for blood circulation when sitting; sit with legs propped up somewhat and out in front with a little bend in them.

Between attempts, massage is good. Use firm circular motions. Try to include tendon attachments with smaller motions. Do not push muscle or tendon over a bone. End up with firm, gentle slapping of area.

Visual Aid

Whoever is your second, another lifter or a coach, have him go through the motion for you slowly. This will make more sense to you than words. Whatever words are used should be simple and meaningful. Your mind should not be cluttered up with a lot of thoughts. You want a few clues to let things happen automatically.

Over-Nervous Lifters

An over-nervous lifter is one who dwells on all the things he is to do and ends up not letting things happen automatically. Sometimes a little time thinking about what you are supposed to do is better than a lot of time. The following has been used successfully. About 4 attempts before, a coach or training partner can manually stretch your knees, wrists, hips, groins and shoulders. This movement will distract you and get your mind off of building up your fears and anxieties. Then with one attempt to go, he can let you concentrate. If you still show too much nervousness before you are to go on the platform, he can shake you up firmly with a hard shake of the shoulders, a hard slap on the rear end or back or even a slap on the face. This is not to be used on just any lifter, but there are some lifters whom no amount of confidence building seems to help. For this type of lifter, something sharp and jolting is often the only distraction from this building up of fears and anxieties.

Things to Have Backstage

Although this is not a complete list, some may think it is too complete. However, just think, when all the hours of training come down to a few precious moments on the platform, you want everything possible available or else all those hours can go down the drain.

paper bag - if you get dizzy, breathe into it

ethyl chloride - for freezing a cramp

smelling salts - for acute awareness before going onto the platform

oxygen - comes in a small bottle; excellent for needed quick recovery, especially for heavier lifters who have to follow themselves on attempts

tape - all sorts, especially $\frac{1}{2}$ inch tape on hand at all times; a change of tape on the thumbs might be needed between warm-ups and often between warm-ups and lifting on the platform

ice chest - ice is always needed for use on such things as injuries and overheated lifters, and also to keep other things cool

vibrator - the ultimate for relaxation and giving a massage

sandpaper - for calluses

file or brush (steel) - for wiping excess chalk off the bar

tape measure - for measuring grip on warm-up bar and platform bar

extra shirt - a change of shirt between the snatch and the clean and jerk gives a fresh feeling

Myoflex - deep rub, enters into blood stream and goes through the kidneys in 30 minutes; not hot

DMSO - if you can get the 90% pure from a doctor, it is great; it acts as a pain reliever and is therapeutic; make sure the skin is clean before you apply it because it takes whatever is on the skin into the body

hot rub - goes well with Myoflex; Myoflex works deep while hot rub gives a good feeling on the surface

Desitin powder - for the thighs instead of chalk; it is finer and works better

chalk - some lifters may forget theirs; don't you!

ice - have a plentiful supply for everything from keeping cool to cramps; take along plastic baggies for applying it, or better yet an ice bag

electrolytes - as a replacement for electrolytes lost during the contest, take pills which contain potassium, magnesium, sodium chloride, phosphorus and the trace elements; during lifting, drink Lytren which is a powder that you mix with water and which can be bought at pharmacies without a prescription

wraps - only legal ones, both ace bandages and knee supports (solid) and anklets, even if you do not normally wear them

scissors, big and little - something always needs to be cut

brine - something may need toughening up

extra weightlifting belt - they do sometimes break!

butterfly bandages, along with other bandages - lifters sometimes crack their chins and cause other such wounds while warming-up; you want something to close a possible wound

injectable electrolytes - when severe cramping takes place, this is the best thing to have on hand; have them administered by a medical person; this may seem too sophisticated, but again, when all the years of training are about to bear fruit, and something goes wrong, you do not want everything to go down the drain

Key Words

Every lifter has some words that key off what he is to do automatically. Know what these words are for you. Make them simple and do not have more than a few. In the heat of competition, only something very basic and meaningful is going to be helpful; the rest will go in one ear and out the other. Some examples are: push hard with the legs; enter in; keep the back at an angle; wait for the popping position; reach up; extend; finish.

Nutrition

When in doubt, eat or drink as little as you are comfortably able. Most of the food will stay and rot in the stomach! Sipping on an electrolyte drink such as Lytren is good. Sipping on coffee or tea is good, and if you like sugar, put some in. Be careful of eating only food with sugar in it; too much sugar will actually cause a drop in sugar that your body can use, and you will begin to feel tired. Something like a little protein broth (meat broth) or half of a high protein candy bar is good to prevent this. Be all means stay away from foods hard to digest (French fries, hamburgers, milk shakes and the like).

2

Selecting Contest Poundages - Marseille-Moscow #1

When the National Coaching Plan was established, our first priority was to make available style, technique and training program information. While we have been successful in doing this, although realizing more needs to be done, we believe now is the time for strong talk about selecting contest poundages. One need only look at the top meets in the United States, especially the Seniors, to know the wrong philosophy is being followed by too many lifters in selecting poundages.

This philosophy which is not working is, simply, whatever is done in training, much more than that is expected from the second attempt. I am not saying that this philosophy does not work with some lifters. All the pressures associated with a contest seem to bring out more than a training session does. Why this is so can only be speculated on. Surely a strong sense of security is one reason. This can be innate or can be developed by going through pressure situations successfully. It can also be developed by constant contact with a good coach.

In talking this over with European coaches, I found that they feel that even among the top flight world competitors there are few athletes who can put on themselves with success the stress and pressure of having to do their best or over their best on their second attempts. Most top flight lifters have developed the ability to cope with stress and pressure by having gone through them successfully, and this means getting in a lot of successful attempts. Does this lead them to mediocre performances? Not in the least. It leads to top performances. To get in a couple of successes before trying one's best or over one's best gives stability so needed for the intense concentration that is necessary to cope with the stress and pressure of lifting equal to or beyond what one has done previously.

I would like to point out some of the pressures which can affect performance. Some are minor, some are major, but all can be major under intense competitive competition. And, again, the majority of the top flight lifters are affected by these pressures. They must be taken into account. If not, a pattern of failure and frustration will develop.

The very act of being judged at a contest is a pressure. It is one thing to do a lift in training where there are no judges, and another to lift under the scrutiny of three judges, especially at high competition where judging seems to be more strict in keeping with international standards. Many lifters know this pressure but do not prepare for it; it becomes magnified when they start too high in poundage.

Another stress is that in training you can take any weight any time you want; in a contest you cannot. You take it when it is your turn, and it may come quicker or later than you want it.

The warm-up platform is different from the contest platform, and this too is a stress. Sometimes it is radically different, but radically or not so radically, it is different and some lifters really get upset over this. In training you lift on only one platform, and you get accustomed to it.

There are often temperature and humidity changes. This can mean over-all difference between your home town and where you are lifting, or it can mean the difference between the warm-up room and the contest area. This is a stress which must be coped with successfully to overcome it. Some lifters do not learn to cope with it successfully, and this particular stress always seems to bother them.

Visual surroundings should be included as a pressure. The open space and different ceiling heights are something to successfully adjust to.

The lifter is lifting with as many as three different makes of bars, the training, warm-up and contest bars. These are sometimes very different bars, especially the way they feel and the hand spacing. Again, it is necessary to learn to cope with this pressure like all the others by going through it successfully in the contest.

Just the fact that a contest means something more than training is pressure. If not gone through successfully, this can blow a lifter's mind in future contests. This means having success with increasing caliber of competition. It is one thing to lift in a small town competition and another to lift in a big city, state, regional, national or even international competition. As one coach put it, "If you can't succeed in your local meet, how are you going to stand the pressure of the World's Championship and succeed? Get in the habit of making only two or three lifts at home and you are either going to bomb out or have to start ridiculously light just to total."

Usually, going along with the increased meaning of the meet is whom you are lifting against. It is one thing to go against Joe Blow and another to go against a top flight competitor about whom you have heard so much and who will give you a tremendous battle. Even though every lifter should know that he should just concentrate on what he is capable of doing and ignore the competition, this is still increased stress and pressure.

Still another stress is what the lifter has done the day of the competition that is different from his routine on a training day when he might have lifted very well. This can range from having to work more on the day of the competition to doing less on the day of competition; both can have an adverse effect. It is usually better to maintain regular daily habits the day of the meet. If you do not, this stress should be taken into account.

The big stress so often not taken into account is weight loss. The body weight during training should not be over the class limit by more than $3\frac{1}{2}$ percent of the class limit. For every pound over this $3\frac{1}{2}$ percent, a weight loss must be taken into account in this manner: from the amount over the class limit $1\frac{1}{4}$ to $1\frac{1}{2}$ pounds per excess pound of body weight should be subtracted from each lift. This would mean, for example, that if a middleweight was weighing 173 pounds during training, he would deduct 12 pounds ($8 \times 1\frac{1}{2}$) from what he did in training on each lift, since 173 is 2 pounds over the $3\frac{1}{2}$ percent allotted limit.

How is weight lost? If a steam or sauna is needed, is the lifter used to it? Not being used to something like a steam bath or sauna can be psychologically draining, if not physically draining. But being used to it removes emotional fear. If weight loss is contemplated, then you should get used to a sauna or steam bath by going in it once or twice a week. There are many ways to lose weight, each with different effects, which is a subject in itself for a long discussion. The main idea I want to point out now is that weight loss is a stress which should be taken into account when the body weight has to drop more than $3\frac{1}{2}$ percent.

Straps should be taken into account. You just cannot go into competition expecting to lift what you did in training when you used straps. It is believed that straps enable a lifter to lift an additional 22 pounds in the snatch alone.

There are countless other stresses and pressures associated with competition. I am far from being a pessimist when I point some of these out. Rather, I am taking into account an aspect of lifting, namely stresses, which should be taken into account when viewing the final goal of lifting the most weight possible in competition. To ignore this is simply not being smart. The pressures and stresses are real to the majority of world class lifters. They are great champions or else they would not be breaking world records like they have been. But in their development, they have learned to cope and respond positively to these stresses and pressures, having gone through the competitive experience successfully many times. To do this means not starting only 5 pounds below their bests or trying their bests on their second attempts. That is too little leeway, too little margin for error. Please do not forget that I am not disregarding the unusual lifter who can start successfully with 5 pounds below his best or at his best and go higher on his second attempt successfully. But he is not the person the majority of lifters should pattern themselves after. If they do, they are fooling themselves, as so many lifters are at present. If this present method worked, I would say to follow it, but it is not working. Too many of our very good top lifters and upcoming lifters are hurting their success by emulating a few distinct lifters. I am not selling the lifter short by advocating that he start lower.

In dealing with what I call the European philosophy of selecting poundages, I would like to point out a few things that should be watched for in the warm-up room which can more accurately give an idea of what poundages to select. It is not enough to say you should start a little lower; more is involved.

The first thing is to have a flexible attitude about starting poundages. Part of the lifter's training should be to practice starting at different weights and taking different jumps in weight. If you are comfortable with this, then your mind will be more flexible about what weights you take and about big or little jumps; you will be ready because you have practiced this in training. You do not want to get locked in on pre-planned starting poundages when the situation is completely different from what you had hoped for.

How the lifter is performing backstage offers some guidelines for choosing his starting poundages. Are you able to control the tempo of your warm-up? You should start slow and slowly build up speed as the weight increases. Controlling tempo means being in control of one's emotions. This is important for conserving energy. From a physiological standpoint and from viewing the Europeans, you should take very few if any power lifts. Hit all snatches and clean and jerks at full position. You may say, "But I can't do 135 like I do 335. I cut my pull." This is not so. With a slow tempo you can hit full position and with perfect coordination, only slower, and with a slow tempo you can conserve energy. There is a tremendous expenditure of energy when moving fast. Why beat 135 to death? It makes for bad movement patterns and expends energy you do not need to expend. Start slow with 135 and hit bottom position. Take a reasonable jump and gradually build your tempo so that your last warm-ups are done with full speed, and you will be ready to lift with good coordination patterns and with lots of energy on the competitive platform.

You want to note your coordination as the warm-ups proceed. One guideline is to have noted when you were "on" at some previous time how much red mark was on your thighs from the bar coming in contact with them. If the mark is more red during the warm-up, then your coordination is off; the weight is being brought in too much or is too jerky. If you are not getting your body to the bar, you will have no red mark, and this is bad because you will be losing leverage. You want a brush, which leaves a slight mark. But brush or not, you want to notice what the mark looks like in comparison to when you were "on" at some previous time.

During your warm-up someone should look at your different body positions as you lift. Are your shoulders in front of the bar as the bar gets to the knees? Is the bar at the same angle when it is at the knees as when it was on the floor? This is an indication not only of coordination but also power in the big muscles of the legs, hips and back. Also, more pertaining to the snatch than to the clean and jerk, are your elbows out to the sides? This is one of the first coordinated movements to go when a lifter is not "on". With elbows to the sides, the lifter gets a good scapula raise; with elbows pointed back, the scapula will not raise nearly as far. Also, more swing at the top will take place.

Another guideline to use backstage for choosing starting poundages is to keep in mind what type of cycle you are in. If it is late in the season, you will have been doing more singles for a longer period of time. If it is early in the season, you will have been doing more reps and less singles. When more singles have been practiced, you can expect more of a difference between a double or triple and a single. When less singles have been practiced and lots of doubles or triples, you can expect less difference between a double or triple and a single.

Still another guideline backstage is how well you are concentrating. It is a well known fact that the more concentration, the more nerve fibers are activated and thus muscle fibers. I believe that the type of concentration needed is pictured clearly by American coach Dick Smith, who said something to the effect that when a photographer takes a picture of a bee on a flower in a field of flowers, he tries to blur out everything but that one bee and that one flower. Relate this to lifting concentration, and I think it illustrates well how intense concentration must be in order to lift heavy weights. Getting back to the original point, how well you are concentrating, I believe honesty should be the rule. Let's face it, not every lifter can get up for every meet. If you cannot concentrate, be human and admit it to yourself; start lower and get something positive out of the meet. And who knows, as you get some success, you might even get into the swing of things. But to start high when not concentrating well is to invite disaster, disaster that can be avoided and a positive experience substituted.

A further clue backstage for your starting poundages is how well you are reacting to the people who are backstage. This is a minor audience. Some lifters capture the attention of other lifters because of the smoothness and cleanness of their lifts. This can turn on the lifter who is being watched. Also, going out onto the platform and making a clean, smooth lift can really turn on a lifter because of audience reaction. By the same token, a lifter cannot get a psychological lift backstage or on stage when his lifts are rugged, sloppy and even missed. Who would respond to this? If you lift smoothly backstage and become inspired by the reaction of others, this probably indicates higher starting poundages; roughness and lack of inspiration indicates lower starting poundages. Likewise, smoothness and good audience reaction when you are on stage may indicate bigger jumps in poundage on succeeding attempts; roughness and poor audience reaction may indicate smaller jumps. I emphasize this audience response; get an audience with a lifter who is lifting smoothly and cleanly, and it will respond and help him. The audience will be silent as he approaches the bar; it will not have to be told to be quiet by the announcer. It will applaud wildly when the lifter completes the lift.

Success in the warm-up room is, of course, a guide to what you should start with. Once in a while, a lifter can have failures in the warm-up room and successfully jump much higher on the platform, but this is the exception, not the rule, and is not to be expected. In my experience watching European lifters, they almost never miss backstage. Everything is a success.

Almost all the European lifters' warm-ups are singles, with only about 6 to 10 of them. By doing singles, you hone in on what is going to be done on the platform, and when I say singles, I mean from 135 on up. It makes no sense to do doubles (refer to the Bulgaria #5 report) when you will be doing a single on the platform. After a good stretch, all that is needed is to sharpen the neuromuscular patterns to be used on the platform. Again, 6 to 10 singles working up from 135 to the starting poundage are all that are necessary.

After your first attempt, what weight should you take next? If you are in good position, especially in the snatch, try to take a weight that is below your best. This takes pressure off you, and you are "building a total". Put pressure on the other guy; force him to take his best or over his best on his second attempt. The snatch is the first lift and should be treated conservatively; more things are apt to go wrong at this time. Be successful in your first two attempts to lay the groundwork for trying whatever weight is needed, within reason, on your third attempt. So many situations can take place that I just want to give one more guideline. Sneak up on the snatch; do not take wild jumps. Even as little as a successful 5 pound increase on the third attempt looks awfully good going into the clean and jerk. Without that increase, it may be a catch-up game which is hard to win. If you want to jump big, do it after the first clean and jerk. By then you have built up a good total in the snatch, and you have totalled with a successful first clean and jerk. Now comes the contest. With 3 or 4 successes under your belt at this stage, you should be set to really pour it on.

If you have to wait around for your lifts, after about three minutes the body starts to cool off. At the end of five minutes, it is really cooling off. Temporary cartilage cells which were initially formed are disappearing. Muscle temperature, muscle contractibility force and muscle flexibility are all going down. Blood is being shunted to other areas. Every three minutes you should be walking around. At the end of five minutes, you should take an 80-85% weight of what you want to do on the next lift and either do a high pull with it or snatch or clean it and then dump it. The idea is to keep warm but to not waste energy. It does not take much energy to pull, but it does to stand up with the weight; this is the reason for dropping the weight after catching it.

I hope that in this discourse I have gotten across the point that the pressure should be taken off our lifters so they can progress faster. This means you should not feel you have to start high on your first attempt and then take your best or over your best on your second attempt. Lifters are under too much pressure when they start so high. There are many pressures to take into account, and I tried to mention a few. These have got to be met successfully in order to go on to bigger lifts. Loss of concentration is seen too often, and it is simply because there is too much pressure.

It is hoped that some of the guidelines to look for backstage will help you select your poundages. The ideas on how to warm up and stay warm should also be of benefit. All these things are designed to help you realize your potential. It is really a wonderful sight to see a lifter, who has learned correct style and has thought out and practiced a good training plan, come to a meet, select wise poundages, make at least 5 of his attempts, set personal records and gain the highest place possible. The rules give the lifter 6 attempts, not 2, so let's make optimum use of them all.

Self-Hypnosis

Although I did not write this, I have used it extensively and feel it belongs in this book. I took this course to use it as an aid to athletes.

SELF-HYPNOSIS CLASS by Stanley G. Kernes, Ph.D.
                          consultant to the 1968 Olympic Women's Diving Team
                          International Academy of Metaphysics, Inc.

SESSION 1

WE AMERICANS are acquainted with HYPNOSIS via the Vaudeville stage. There is a vast difference between the techniques used in stage and medical hypnosis. One uses FORCE, the other, COOPERATION. Perhaps these forceful techniques used by our early stage hypnotists (usually resulting in embarrassing situations) tainted hypnosis to such a degree that the many benefits to be derived from it have not been brought to the notice of the general public.

HYPNOSIS integrates and stimulates the brain to perform SPECIALIZED TASKS in a way that the conscious mind cannot understand.
The application of ANESTHETICS and SLEEP to an individual will produce a change in the brain waves (rhythms). HYPNOSIS does not produce any change in the brain waves, so consequently it <u>does</u> <u>not</u> put the brain to sleep.

THE NEXT logical step for man to take is to learn to expand his own mental powers through the use of HYPNOSIS and SELF-HYPNOSIS. The new tool could very well gain personal success for each of you and open many new doors: for instance, learning depends on the <u>power of the Brain to recall</u> or RECOVER what is ALREADY known. Recovering this tremendous quantity of information from the brain by the use of CONSCIOUS WILL POWER is usually difficult....however, through the use of Hypnosis, this information can not only be recalled easier, but also retained.

Let us take a case of INSOMNIA. Sleep induced by hypnosis has advantages which far outweigh those of DRUG INDUCED sleep, for hypnosis functions not by physically toxifying the brain centers to produce the unconscious, but by relieving the PSYCHOLOGICAL TENSION which is at the root of the symptom.

ONE OF the biggest misconceptions about Hypnosis which should be corrected is that a person who is hypnotized must be unconscious. In fact, nothing could be further from the truth, because even in the deepest trance, the SUBJECT can hear the doctor. He can answer questions and will always know what is going on. This is so true, that as a doctor, I always explain to my patients the signs that indicate he or she is in a Hypnotic State (breathing), otherwise they would deny that they were hypnotized, because they are perfectly aware of EVERYTHING THAT OCCURRED. Only in an extremely deep state could loss of this awareness occur. This state is <u>not</u> reached by Self-Hypnosis, but usually by a professional Hypnotist applying the proper techniques to a CONDITIONED PATIENT.

The word HYPNOTISM, although it has played its part in HUMAN LIFE since the existence of man, has only been used for a little over a hundred years. Witch doctors, Medicine men and priests have all practiced it.

MODERN MEDICAL HYPNOSIS can be said to have started nearly 200 years ago in SWITZERLAND. This was the start of FAITH CURES, which were used by Father Gassner when he discovered he had such powers of healing. Today these same principles are applied scientifically.

FRANZ ANTON HESMER, a young German physician was so impressed with Father Gassner's work, that he carried his theories further in a way as to apply it to the importance of the fact that mental treatment can have a DIRECT BEARING on the ILLNESS OF THE BODY, and that its proper use can be of immense benefit to mankind.

England's John Elliotson, along with James Braid, were very progressive in the use of Hypnosis, being concerned with both PSYCHOLOGICAL and PHYSIOLOGICAL problems.

AND THEN THERE WAS FREUD....AND CARL JUNG....

HYPNOTIC STATE	The person in a HYPNOTIC STATE is self-absorbed as in a FANTASY... It can be compared to a dream-like state. SUBJECT is fully aware of what is happening and extremely alert.
WHY DOES HYPNOSIS WORK?	Most all human beings are suggestible and suggestion is the key to Hypnotism.
CONDITIONING	You are to be conditioned to the PROPER TECHNIQUES OF SELF-HYPNOSIS, using the key word "BLUE ROSE". Blue Rose will condition a response to your being able to relax to a deep state.
SELF-HYPNOSIS	This is a natural form of relaxation which makes it easier for the individual to discover and understand the workings of his BODY and MIND.....Learn to control the factors causing your distress. It assists the individual in becoming "EMOTIONALLY SELF-SUSTAINING".
CLINICAL HYPNOSIS (Hypnotherapy)	Relaxing the patient properly to reach the subconscious mind so that beneficial suggestions can take effect. These suggestions, when given over and over, can change the emotional and physical make-up of the individual. (Do not confuse with stage hypnosis)...

THE CONSCIOUS MIND...INTELLECTUAL MIND...OBJECTIVE MIND...RULER OF OUR MENTAL WORLD

10% of our MIND	This is the part of the mind with which we perceive, reason, judge and reject. By the operation of the conscious mind, we are AWARE of our power to think, to know, to will and to choose. Through the conscious mind, we have conscious communications with every part of our body and respond to every sensation of SIGHT, SOUND, SMELL, TASTE, AND FEELING.

The conscious mind <u>controls</u> the subconscious mind by thoughts. Thoughts are influenced by your environment. If your thoughts are bad, either change your thoughts or change your environment.

THE SUBCONSCIOUS MIND.....SUBJECTIVE MIND

90% of our MIND	This is the part of the mind which presides over all the INVOLUNTARY PROCESSES OF YOUR BODY, SUCH AS digestion, assimilation, elimination, the beating of your heart, the circulation of your blood, and the secretions, which are manufactured by various glands. It is the STOREHOUSE OF MEMORY, the SEAT OF HABIT AND INSTINCT, the CENTER OF EMOTIONS, and its action is automatic.

It is like a four or five year old child, with VERY MUCH POWER, but has to be told OVER and OVER AGAIN. It will work out the suggestion you give to it to the end...as IT understands it...so keep the suggestions simple so that a four or five year old child could understand.

THE SUBCONSCIOUS MIND takes everything said to it literally and works out the problem as it sees it. Remember...the subconscious cannot take a joke. Whatever you tell it, it will begin to work out the problem as it is understood by the subconscious mind.

YOUR PRESENT CHARACTER is made up of countless thoughts, beliefs, habits...entertained and formed by you in the past. This character is impressed on your subconscious mind and is the cause of your present health, your present state of mind, and your present financial status. If you wish to change all or any of the above mentioned, the AFFIRMATION to follow will be very effective.

AFFIRMATION: I AM HEALTHY, STRONG, YOUNG, POWERFUL, LOVING, HARMONIOUS,
                 SUCCESSFUL AND HAPPY.

THE EFFECTIVENESS IS BROUGHT about when a statement is continuously made by the CONSCIOUS MIND and accepted by the SUBCONSCIOUS MIND as a pattern by which to weave your future. Your present conditions are the result of your past thinking. You will be what you are thinking today.

Man is the highest expression of individual life because he THINKS. Sometimes we tend to blame others for our misfortunes, but the fact remains, we are entirely responsible for our success or failure, happiness or misery. MAN makes himself, creates his own personality, character and circumstances.

IN OTHER WORDS:

Destiny is fixed by our subconscious actions. You are not a slave to circumstances. You are the CREATOR of your own destiny...we attract to ourselves only that which corresponds to our subconscious impressions, and you can always make a new start by changing your subconscious impressions.

So...if you have THOUGHT FAILURE...THINK SUCCESS. Replace sick thoughts with thoughts of health. If there is any reason for unhappiness, resolve to put it out of your mind for in this case...LIKE ATTRACTS LIKE, and the more you think discordant conditions, the more such conditions will manifest for you.

REMEMBER...it is necessary to concentrate on what you WANT. When you do think, you are impressing that desire on your subconscious mind. NEVER let your thoughts dwell on what you DO NOT WANT.

It is extremely important, even though it might seem that everything is going against us, and since we are creatures of habit, this makes it that much harder when we try to change. Remember, if you want to change your course when driving a car, you might have to stop, back up, go forward and maybe go back again before you get turned around. In changing the impressions and habits of our subconscious minds we could experience some difficulty...so always believe what you desire as accomplished fact.

INSTRUCTIONS

SELECT a place reasonably quiet, where there will definitely not be any interruptions. If there is a phone nearby, TAKE IT OFF THE RECEIVER SO IT WILL NOT RING.

Make sure your pets (and/or children) are not around to bother you. Your clothing should be loose, so the circulation of the blood can flow freely. Tight shoes and watchbands should also be removed. Later on, when you are conditioned to BLUE-ROSE, this is not as necessary, as the effectiveness overrides those factors. The room should be dark, or at least as dark as possible. Again, this will not make that much difference later on, but for the present, darkness is recommended.

TURN ON FAN...MOTOR...HAIRDRYER...BLOWER...NOISEMAKER

Lie down on your back...feet stretched out straight (do not cross) - arms down at your side (do not fold). Lay there about one minute and just relax. Flex each muscle..starting at your toes and working up to your head.

TAKE A DEEP BREATH...LET IT OUT SLOWLY, CLOSING YOUR EYES AT THE SAME TIME... AND THINK TO YOURSELF SLOWLY:

"BLUEROSE" - I am relaxing. I am relaxing more and more...It feels so good just to let go...Just to let every muscle go limp. Every muscle, every nerve and every nerve ending is relaxing more and more now, and I'm drifting deeper, deeper, down and down...feeling so good and so relaxed now and I am drifting even deeper and going down and down and relaxing more and more. I feel so relaxed and every nerve and muscle is relaxing more and more now.

Every nerve and every muscle in my face is relaxing more and more...every nerve and every muscle in the back of my neck - the side of my neck - down my back and around is relaxing more and more now. All the tension in the back of my neck is draining down and out of my body harmlessly...I am relaxing more and more now. Every nerve and every muscle in my shoulders, (repeat every nerve and every muscle in my..) arms...hands...chest...stomach...pelvic area...thighs ...legs...feet, are more and more relaxed now.

From the top of my head, to the tip of my toes, I am completely relaxed and I am drifting even deeper and deeper and going down and down, deeper and deeper, down and down to very deep and relaxing, easy, easy sleep. I feel so relaxed now...NOTHING AND NO ONE can bother or disturb me...all my fears and all my doubts and all my guilt are draining down and out of my mind harmlessly. My mind is quiet and calm...and I have a feeling of inner peace, inner harmony. Every day I am thinking more and more positively. Every day I am thinking in a more positive way. I reject all negative thoughts, words and vibrations. Every day I am becoming more and more positive in both body and mind. My attitude towards everything and everyone is getting better and better and no one and nothing can bother or disturb me in any negative sense. Every day I am becoming more and more confident in myself and my ability to perform.

COUNT TO THREE AND SAY AS YOU COUNT:

1 - My mind is becoming more and more alert.

2 - I am waking up and my mind is more alert.

3 - Eyes wide open.

SECTION V

TRAINING AIDS

Pain Relief

There is a transcutaneous nerve stimulation device that was used very successfully at the Olympics in Montreal. It is called Neoromod, and it is put out by Medtronic, Inc. (3055 Old Highway Eight, Minneapolis, Minnesota 55418). What it does is pass small electrical currents through the skin. These currents depolarize nerves which carry pain feelings.

The Neuromod has two uses. One, it acts in place of drugs to relieve immediate pain so that athletic activity can continue. Two, it is useful in cases where the injury is old and chronic. In both cases, it lets the inflamed nerves rest and recover. Pain initially tells you to slow down, something is wrong. But then, many times after things are healed, pain persists and serves no useful function. The nerves have just remained inflamed.

To go to a physical therapist who has one of these devices costs approximately $5.00 to $7.50 per treatment, and it takes 3 to 6 treatments for results to show. Sometimes it takes longer. It is useful to know that these units are available from some pharmacists and usually rent for about $60 per month. Sometimes an even longer period of time than a month is needed for good results. In such a case and for use with future injuries, buying such a unit may be considered. The same pharmacist will sell a Neuromod for between $340 and $375. In order to use a Neuromod at a physical therapist's or to rent or buy one, a doctor's prescription is needed.

If something is structurally wrong and surgery is not wanted, using this device may permit athletic activity. Using it two times a day for between one and two hours is what is usually recommended. Since it attaches to a shirt pocket, work can be done while wearing it.

Increasing Circulation

Although I did not write this, I have used it extensively and feel it belongs in this book.

INCREASING CIRCULATION-----WITH COLD!   by A. G. Edwards, M.A.
                                          Assistant Athletic Trainer
                                          United States Air Force Academy

It has long been the feeling that the best method (if not the only one) of increasing circulation to a body part is through the application of heat. Only in recent years, and with work such as The Rehabilitation Center in Vallejo, California, is doing with ice, has this theory been questioned.

The penetrative effects of heat have been found to only reach a depth of one-sixteenth to one-eighth inch; whereas, the effects of temperature change with cold have been recorded to bone level.

A limb immersed in a bath at 105.8° F. showed subcutaneous temperature rise of 7.2° (93.2° - 100.4° F.) in approximately twenty-five minutes and remained at that level for ninety minutes. A deep muscle temperature rise of only 1.8° (96.8° - 98.6° F.) was reached in approximately thirty minutes and remained at that level for ninety minutes. A limb immersed in a bath at 59.0° F. showed a subcutaneous temperature drop of 27.0° (93.2° - 66.2° F.) in thirty minutes, 32.4° (93.2 - 60.8° F.) in sixty minutes, and 36.0° (93.2° - 57.2° F.) in ninety minutes. The deep muscle decrease in temperature was recorded at 21.6° (98.6° - 77.0° F.) in thirty minutes, and 32.4° (98.6° - 66.2° F.) in ninety minutes.

We can see by the preceding paragraph that the external application of cold is more penetrating and has greater effect on both subcutaneous and deep muscle tissue. Bierman and Friedlander in their study, "Penetrative Effects of Cold", show that cold penetrates more deeply than most forms of heat.

If you now accept the hypothesis that cold is more penetrating and has a greater effect on tissue, then you must be asking yourself, "Is the effect beneficial to increasing circulation?" If cold is applied for a period of time ranging from ten to thirty minutes, there is a vasoconstriction and decreased blood flow. For a period of time ranging from thirty to sixty minutes after application of cold.

Only during the application of heat are vasodilation and increased blood flow present. Immediately upon the removal of the application of heat there is a reflex vasoconstriction, hence the increased blood flow is reduced. A reflex vasodilatation is the reaction to the removal of cold application. These reflex reactions are realized because of the protective mechanisms of the body. Dr. George Thosteson stated in his August 4, 1970 column in the Colorado Springs, Colo. SUN that "Your body diverts circulation in response to needs. For example, your face gets red in cold weather because more circulation is drawn to the exposed skin surface to warm them". All of us have experienced cold, red, throbbing ears after periods of cold exposure. Can you remember the long time that warmth could be felt in the ears and the throbbing of the blood flow through them?

The same physical changes that applications of heat produce, for only the length of application and for only one-sixteenth to one-eighth inch below the surface of the skin, are produced throughout the subcutaneous and deep muscle tissue for thirty to sixty minutes, when cold applications are applied.

FASTER RESPONSE

A faster and more efficient response to the application of cold can also be attributed to the fact that the Krause (cold) sensory receptors are less deeply planted in the tissue and there are eight times more Krause receptors than Ruffini (hot) receptors.

A by-product to the increased blood flow through the application of cold is the local anesthesia produced. This allows for pain-free range of motion of the part. Thomas Gucker states, "Even a 100 per cent increase in muscle blood flow produced by heat is small compared with that resulting from activity produced by voluntary muscular contraction or even by electric stimulation."

Other physical changes produced by increased blood flow are relaxation of muscle spasm, nutrition, healing, and the carrying off of waste and edema. Also, Downey points out that the rate of cell metabolism increases as the temperature increases. When cold is applied the cell metabolism decreases. One of the products of cell metabolism is lactic acid. Therefore, the application of heat to remove excess metabolites might in fact produce more unwanted lactic acid.

Mead and Knott report success in reducing spasticity by the use of cold applications in such conditions as quadriplegia, arthritis, and poliomyelitis. Viel found that patients that had cerebral vascular accidents, multiple sclerosis, and traumatic quadriplegia experienced relief from spasticity of the finger, wrist, and ankle flexor groups after cold applications. Hayden reported the early results of treatment of acute and painful skeletal muscular conditions with ice massage. In this program 1000 patients were treated with ice massage. Eight hundred and fifty of the patients returned to military duty within one hour following treatment. Only three of this group required an advanced form of treatment.

Grant later reported a continuation of Hayden's work. Seven thousand patients were treated with ice massage. He states that satisfactory results were achieved in over 80 percent of the patients and that less than five percent of the patients required more than six treatments. Juvenal has reported success in using Grant's method of ice massage in the treatment of athletic injuries.

The author has used ice therapy with especially good results on joints such as the ankle, knee, shoulder, and elbow. Having practiced all except one year in the field of athletic rehabilitation, it is imperative to obtain the maximum responses in a minimum time. Ice therapy has produced the desired effects through faster, longer, more efficient blood flow.

Measure Those Training Lifts
With A Few Pieces of Wood, A Piece of String
A Nail, and Rubber Bands

How many times have you pulled training weights higher than need be when you knew you only wanted to pull them to the height needed to clean or snatch contest weights? How many times have you wanted to jerk a weight only as high as needed to jerk big poundages but found you did not know if you were jerking the weight too high? How many times did you not know if you were jerking the weight straight up or not?

The answers to the above questions are probably "many times" and "I don't know". These need not be the answers. With a few pieces of wood, a piece of string, a nail, and rubber bands, you can tell if you are pulling the weight to the needed height, jerking the weight a certain height or jerking the weight straight up.

To make the equipment which will help you, nail a thin piece of wood at a right angle to a thicker, long piece of wood which, in turn, has been nailed at a right angle to a flat piece of wood for support. To see if the jerk is going straight, or if the pull is being pulled straight, hang a piece of string from the horizontal thin piece of wood. To stabilize the string, tie a nail to the end of it. Have a coach or training partner place this apparatus near you and put the string in line with the path the bar will take. It is then easy to see if the bar is jerked or pulled straight.

To see if you are pulling or jerking the bar to the needed height, find out the height that you need and then put a mark at this height on the long vertical piece of wood. At this mark attach a string of rubber bands, made by tying together a package of small rubber bands. The apparatus is placed behind you and directly behind the sleeve of the bar. When you lift, your training partner or coach stretches the string of rubber bands out to the front and side of you - directly in front of the sleeve of the bar. If the bar is pulled or jerked above the marked height, it hits the rubber bands and will stretch them upward. In this way you know exactly if the bar reached the height you wanted or went beyond.

This apparatus can also be used to measure your high pulls. Many times a lifter will want to pull the bar to just above the belt for a clean pull or to some higher height for a snatch pull. He will make his high pull with a certain weight to the desired height and then fail with that weight in a contest. Why does this happen? This could be because when he was practicing his high pull in training, he was bending his knees so that what then appeared to be a high pull to the desired height was really a lower pull. With this apparatus, you can bend your knees but know exactly if you pulled the bar to the needed height for a clean or snatch.

One final note is that you should use rubber bands and not rope or string in making this device. The rubber bands will stretch and not break or bother the liftor, whereas a rope or string might break or get in the way.

4

Timing the Speed of the Bar

At the 1976 AAU Weightlifting Convention in Phoenix, Arizona, I gave a presentation of an inexpensive (made for under $175) device for measuring the speed of the bar. The top weightlifting countries of the world are doing this measuring for good reason but with much more costly apparatus. This particular device that I presented was designed to be within the price range of any weightlifting enthusiast.

The top countries in the weightlifting world are using time measuring devices because once the speed of a successful limit lift is known, training lifts should approximate this speed much of the time. This is because of neuromotor specificity, and the proportion of fast twitch and slow twitch muscle fibers which is developed for a particular athletic event. For this same reason, pulling squats should also be done at the speed of a limit lift. I will not go into the details of neuromotor specificity and fast and slow twitch muscle fibers because I have explained them in other articles. Rather, I would like to give a brief practical guide to the use of the timing device.

The timer is calibrated in hundredths of a second. Thousandths of a second can be used, but this would be much more expensive. Timers calibrated in tenths of a second are cheaper but not accurate enough. Thus, the practical one to use is one measuring in hundredths of a second.

Wires connect the timing device to the transformer and the relays. The wires that go to the bar are tied around a hook so that the length of the wire that is free to travel straight up from the floor to the bar is constant and can be changed to different constants.

What happens is that the bar rests on a switch mat. When the bar leaves the switch mat, the timer goes on. When the bar reaches the desired height, the wires which are attached to the wing nut of the collar pull off and the timer goes off. The timer is read and then reset.

It is somewhat of an inconvenience to time all lifts because the wires after pulling off the wing nut of the collar have to be clamped on again. In addition, with every lift being timed, a lifter can become stale with too much exactness demanded. It becomes practical then to time just once a week and only with weights 80% and above.

I believe the timing of the bar to be of the utmost importance. Too many lifters are not doing 80%+ lifts at the speed with which they would do a successful limit lift, they are not doing pulls at limit lift speed, and they are not doing pull squats at limit lift speed. Therefore, much of their practice is not preparing them for what they want to do. It is important that much of the lifter's practice be at speeds used in competition.

Also, the timing of the bar is needed for psychological reasons. Having as his only incentive increasing the weight on the bar brings staleness and boredom to the lifter's training. It is refreshing for the lifter to once in a while use time as an incentive.

Two pictures follow on the next page to show the timing device which I presented in Phoenix and to show it being used.

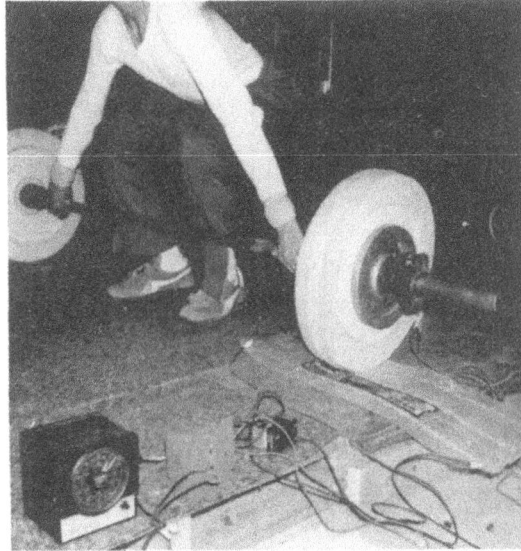

#1 Note electrical timer, transformer and
relays all lined up. Also note the
measured wire attached by clips to the
wing nut of the collar. The plastic
switch mat, on which the bar is resting,
has wires running through it.

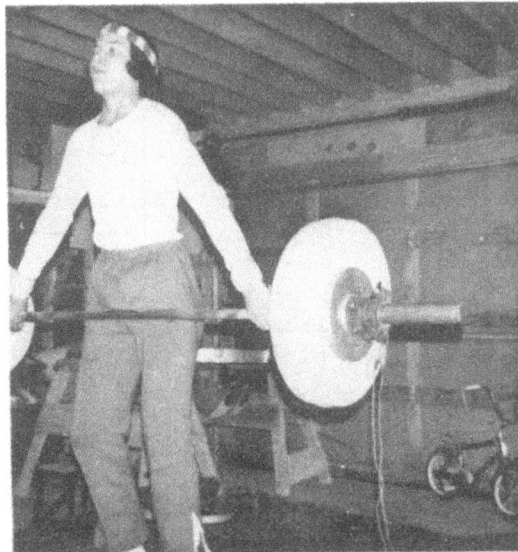

#2 The lifter is just about at the top of
his pull. The length of the wire is
measured so that when the top of the
pull is reached, the clips pull off the
wing nut.

Equipment Schedule

1. GE #RT1 35VA 120/30Volt Transformer
2. Cutler-Hammer #9575H2524-66 Relay - 24Volt Coil
3. Cutler-Hammer #9575H2441-66 Relay - 24Volt Coil
4. GE. 24Volt Pilot Light with Green Lense
5. Ademco #158. 30"Wide Switch Mat.
6. Mueller Alligator Clips - 2 Req'd.
7. Copper Contact Plate on Barbell Plate Collar
8. Singer Electronic Elapsed Time Indicator

Operating Instructions

1. Plug in cord to 120v source (leads 6) not connected
2. Reset Clock
3. Place Weight on to Mat 5
4. Green Pilot 4 on
5. Attach leads 6 to plate 7
6. Lift weight - time on clock is weight off mat to disconnect
7. Record Reading of Clock
8. Repeat steps 2,3,4,5,6,7
9. Unplug cord when finished.

120 V A.C.

30V A.C.

120V A.C.

Schematic Drawing

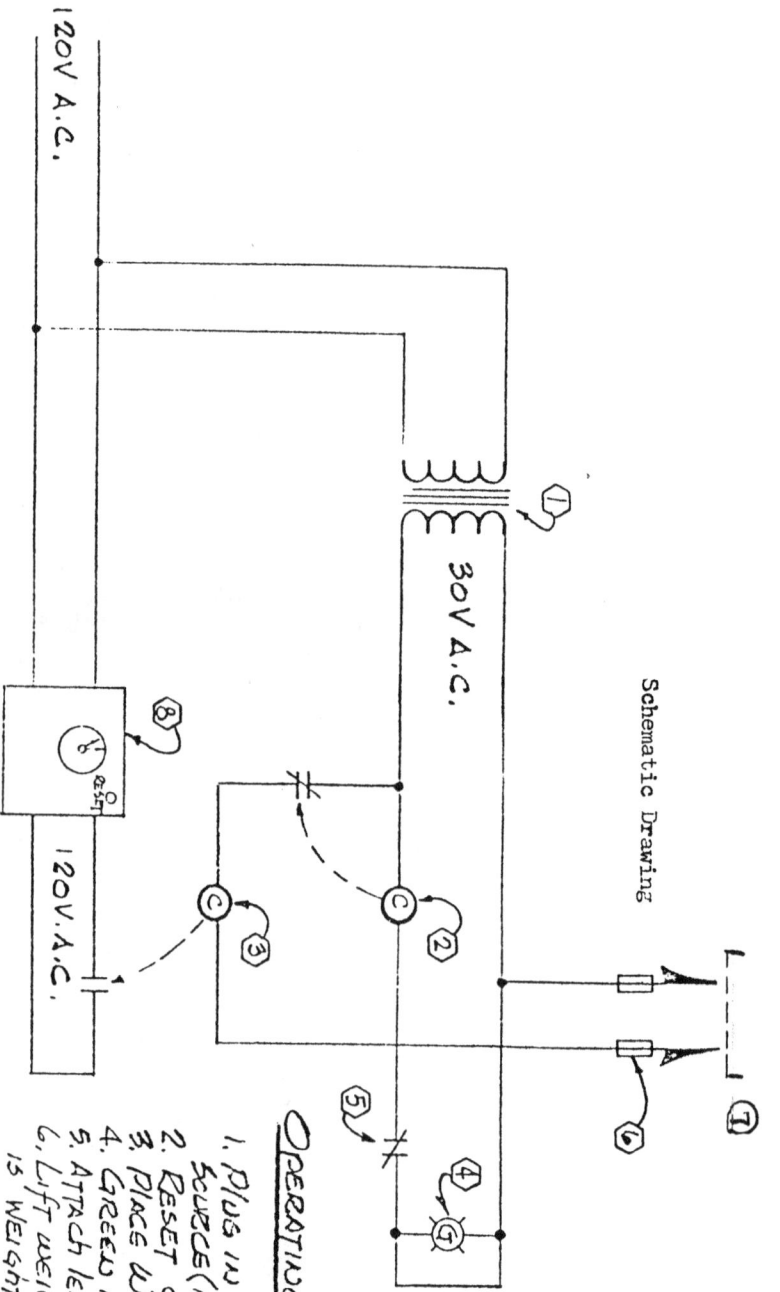

R.W. Bybee —
Bybee Engineering,
Santa Fe NM 10-7-76
FE

110

5

Magic Circle

In the Marseille-Moscow #2 (Leg Work) article, I described an apparatus called the Magic Circle, put out by Iron Man Industries. I feel the need to explain more fully the use of this equipment because of the great importance I believe it carries. (Please remember, I receive no financial remuneration from Iron Man Industries for the sale of Magic Circles.)

The Magic Circle's greatest value is that it can be used for "pulling squats" (squats that simulate the double knee bend style of pull; see the Specialized Pull leg exercises in Marseille-Moscow #2). If you look at the pictures at the end of this article, you will see the lifter is squatting as he does for the double knee bend. In picture #1, the bar would be around the floor level with the shoulders directly above or a little ahead of the bar. As the bar would come to the knees (picture #2), the shoulders would go well in front of the bar. Then the lifter scoops under as when doing the double knee bend (picture #3) and then uses his hips and his legs to extend straight up as he would do when pulling (picture #4).

This action is easy with the Magic Circle because as the shoulders go in front of the bar, the Magic Circle is pulled back toward the body (see the difference in distance the front part of the Magic Circle is from the lifter's body in pictures #1 and #2, and note that the front edge has been pulled toward the body), and the lifter remains in good balance. With a bar on the shoulders, this cannot be done without extreme pressure on the lower back and discomfort of the shoulders. When a lifter does this type of pulling squat, he gets a lot of transference of power that is gained from squatting; the power is transferred to pulling. It is a physiological fact that the greatest transference of power from progressive resistance exercises to the specific action done in any given sport takes place when both actions are as similar to each other as possible.

Another value of the Magic Circle is having a lot of weight feel comfortable on the shoulders. This is very important for beginners. Leg and hip power is so important, but beginners shy away from gaining it in the form of one of the best exercises, squats, because of the bar digging into the shoulders. Even with pads, it can still be uncomfortable and cumbersome.

A final value is the safety of handling large weights when nobody else is there. The hands can be put on the thighs, and with a hard push by the hands, the lifter will come right up (see picture #5).

So with its comfort, safety when handling heavy weights, and its ability to be used effectively when doing "pulling squats", the Magic Circle is something which can certainly help an Olympic lifter.

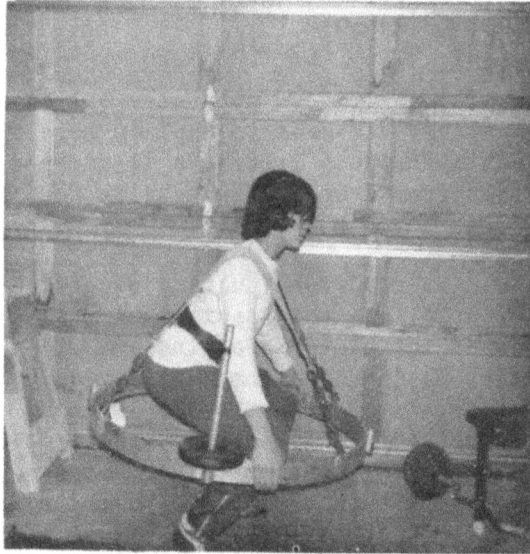

#1 The bar would be around floor level
with the shoulders directly above or
a little in front of the bar.

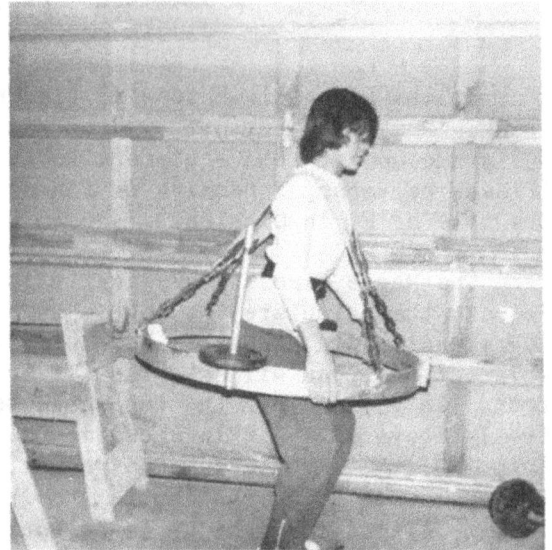

#2 The bar would be around the knees with
the shoulders well in front of the bar.

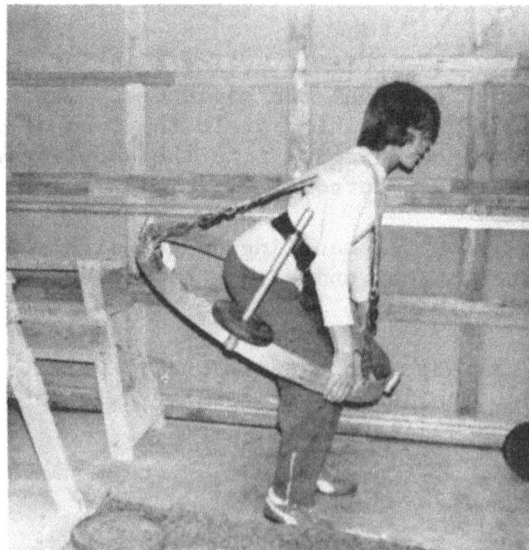

#3 The lifter has scooped under like he
would when doing a pull.

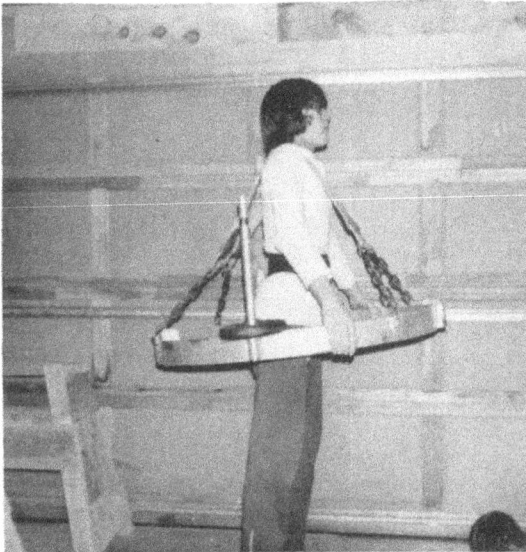

#4 The lifter has extended straight up as he would when doing a pull.

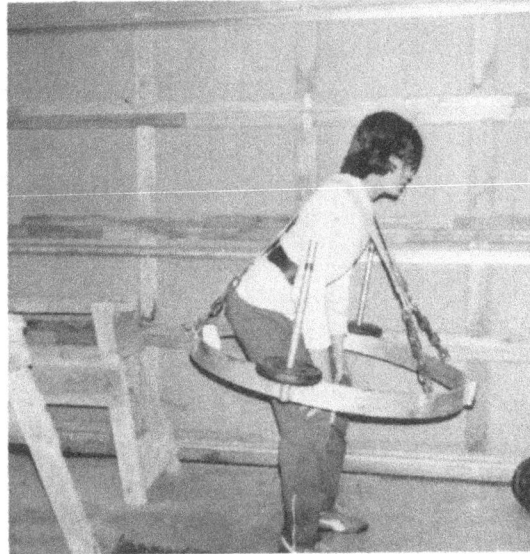

#5 The lifter puts his hands on his thighs to help himself up from a heavy squat.

SECTION VI

NUTRITION

1

Brief Summary of Some Nutrients

Protein

Purpose: to maintain and produce body cells

Deficiency Symptoms: fatigue, bad digestion, inadequate enzyme action, undergrowth, inadequate body acid-base balance, susceptibility to disease

Foods High in Complete Protein: organ meats, muscle meats, yeast, milk, milk products, soybeans, eggs, fish, fowl

Remarks: A protein has to be complete (containing all 8 essential amino acids) to be able to be used or stored. Two or more incomplete proteins eaten at the same meal may form a complete protein.

Fat

Purpose: forms part of every cell, permits valuable intestinal bacteria to multiply, forms sex and adrenal hormones, helps regulate water balance, transports vitamins A, D, E and K to the cells, acts as a homogenizing agent that lets tiny particles of fat and cholesterol pass readily into the tissues

Deficiency Symptoms: dry hair, fatigue, sterility, loss of sex interest, overweight or underweight, bloatedness

Foods High in Essential Fatty Acids: French dressing, mayonnaise, salad oil, cottonseed oil, avocados, nuts

Remarks: For fat to work, the essential fatty acids (linoleic, linolenic and arachidonic acids) should be present in the fat eaten.

Vitamin A

Purpose: day and night vision, skin and mucous membrane maintenance, development of bones and tooth enamel, good appetite, normal digestion, reproduction, lactation, formation of red and white blood corpuscles, prenatal development

Deficiency Symptoms: eyestrain, roughness and dryness of skin, blackheads, bronchial infections

Foods High in Vitamin A: fish-liver oils, liver, egg yolks, butter, cream, carrots, green vegetables, yellow vegetables

Remarks: The quality of vitamin A in foods is related to their intensity of color.

Vitamin B Complex

Purpose: energy production, stress combator, hair and skin maintenance, proper HCl and other digestive juice secretions, blood vessel and eye maintenance

Deficiency Symptoms: lack of energy and coordination, thinning of hair, clogged arteries, nervous disorders, eye strain, incomplete digestion, broken and weak capillaries

Foods High in Vitamin B Complex: liver, yeast, converted rice, wheat germ, whole grains and breads and cereals

Remarks: The vitamin B complex must be taken in the right proportion; too much of one or more of the vitamin B's causes an inbalance which will create a deficiency in one or more of the other vitamin B's. The B vitamins grow best in the intestine on milk sugar and fatty acids. HCl acid is needed for their absorption.

Vitamin C

Purpose: wards off colds and infections, maintains blood vessels, strengthens bones, helps in healing wounds and injuries, acts as a hydrogen acceptor in carbohydrate metabolism, helps normal vision, combats stress

Deficiency Symptoms: repeated and long colds, fatigue, slow recovery from injuries, easily bruised, poor vision
Foods High in Vitamin C: citrus fruits, green vegetables, tomatoes
Remarks: Vitamin C and calcium work together; vitamin C without calcium does little good. The sweeter the orange, the higher the vitamin C content is. Natural vitamin C is destroyed by heat. Cigarettes destroy vitamin C readily.

Vitamin D

Purpose: aids in absorption of calcium, helps prevent tooth decay, helps bone calcification
Deficiency Symptoms: bad teeth and weak bones, vitamin C and calcium deficiencies
Foods High in Vitamin D: fish liver oils, artificially produced vitamin D in milk
Remarks: It is hard for the body to produce vitamin D.

Vitamin E

Purpose: forms part of an enzyme which helps utilize fat; protects essential fatty acids, vitamins A and B complex, and the pituitary, adrenal and sex hormones from being destroyed by oxygen
Deficiency Symptoms: all symptoms associated with the lack of all the nutrients it protects (fatty acids, vitamin A and vitamin B complex), especially fatigue
Foods High in Vitamin E: wheat germ and wheat germ oil, whole grain breads and cereals
Remarks: Ninety percent of vitamin E is lost in deep-frying. The American diet is very low in vitamin E.

Calcium

Purpose: aids in transportation of nerve impulses, is necessary for vitamin C to work, aids in normal activity during menstruation, acts as a pain killer, is necessary for the clotting of blood, works with vitamin D for good skeletal and dental health
Deficiency Symptoms: irritability, vitamin C deficiency symptoms, abnormal pain during menstruation, cramping
Foods High in Calcium: milk and milk products, green vegetables
Remarks: Good HCl content in the stomach is necessary for calcium absorption; however, even when HCl is adequate, a glass of orange juice or milk aids calcium digestion. Concentrated carbohydrates decrease calcium absorption. Too much or too little fat decreases calcium absorption. No more than twice as much phosphorus as calcium should be taken. Calcium lactate or calcium gluconate are good sources of calcium. Extra calcium should be taken if lots of meat and wheat germ or whole grains are eaten.

Iron

Purpose: needed for hemoglobin and nuclei in all body cells
Deficiency Symptoms: anemia, fatigue
Foods High in Iron: liver, kidneys, yeast, wheat germ, whole grains and breads, muscle meats
Remarks: HCl must be adequate for iron absorption. Natural sources of iron are better than iron salts; vitamin C is destroyed when iron salts are used.

Trace Minerals

Cobalt, Copper, Zinc, Manganese, Flourine
Purpose: mainly to form part of the enzyme systems of the body
Deficiency Symptoms: related to insufficient enzyme action
Foods High in Trace Minerals: whole grains and breads and cereals, sea foods

Remarks: Split stalks, cracked cores and uneven ripening are symptoms of lack of
          trace minerals in vegetables.

Phosphorus

Remarks: This is easy to get in an American diet.

Potassium

Purpose: has to do with nerve conduction and body fluid balance
Foods with Potassium: whole grains, cereals and breads, vegetables
Deficiency Symptoms: nervousness, insomnia, slow growth, cramping

Magnesium

Purpose: needed in action of 30 enzymes
Deficiency Symptoms: irritability, nervousness
Foods with Magnesium: whole grains and breads, vegetables
Remarks: The requirement should be half of calcium required.

High Nutrition in Foods

I stress the importance of a good, well-balanced diet. You may want to give some foods added nutrition by adding some nutritious things to them. The following are all examples of extra nutritious recipes.

Pancakes

Hi-Protein Egg Pancakes

3 eggs
1/4 cup high protein powder
1/2 cup fresh milk
3 tbsp non-fat dry milk
2 tbsp wheat germ oil
1/8 tsp salt

Pre-heat oven to 450°. Butter a 10 inch pie tin or skillet and place in refrigerator while preparing the ingredients. In a blender or electric mixer, beat the eggs while gradually adding high protein, milk, dry milk, wheat germ oil and salt. Beat and mix thoroughly. Pour into the cold, buttered pan and place in oven for 10 minutes. Then reduce heat to 350° and bake for 10 minutes more, or until puffed and brown. For breakfast or dinner serve with lean bacon, ham, sausage or liver. For an-all in-one lunch and dessert add 2 tablespoons honey to the batter before mixing. Serve with applesauce.

Hi-Protein Ranch Pancakes

1/4 cup pancake mix
1/2 cup high protein powder
1 cup whole milk
2 tbsp wheat germ oil

Mix up pancakes and cook on griddle. Fry four eggs. On a plate place layers of pancakes alternated with eggs. Top with honey.

Cookies

Brownies

1/2 cup honey
1/2 cup wheat germ oil
1/2 cup high protein powder
2 eggs, beaten
1 1/3 cups oat flour
1/3 cup rice flour
1/2 cup chopped nuts
1 tsp vanilla extract

Blend honey, wheat germ oil and high protein. Gradually add eggs. Mix well. Stir in flour. Add nuts and vanilla. Pour into greased 8" x 8" pan. Bake at 350° for 25-30 minutes. When cool, cut into squares and serve.

High Protein Cookies

1 cup sugar
1 cup honey
1 cup butter
2 eggs, beaten
1 tsp soda
1 tsp ginger
2 1/2 cups flour
1 1/2 cups high protein powder

Pre-heat oven to 400°. Cream sugar, honey and butter. Add eggs. Sift flour, soda, ginger and high protein and add to other mixture. Drop by spoonfulls onto cookie sheet and bake until cookies are golden brown.

For variety,
Optional: 1/2 cup chopped raisins, nuts, dates, etc.

Chocolate Drop Cookies

2 cups sugar
1/4 cup margarine
1/4 cup cocoa
1/2 cup milk

Mix sugar, margarine, cocoa and milk in saucepan; bring to boil quickly. Reduce heat to medium and boil 3 or 4 minutes or until a little dropped into cold water forms a soft ball (234°). Remove from

Chocolate Drop Cookies (cont.)

   ½ cup unsaturated peanut butter
   1 tsp vanilla
   3 cups oats, mixed with:
   ½ cup wheat germ

heat and stir in peanut butter and vanilla. Stir in oats-wheat germ mixture. Drop by teaspoonfuls onto waxed paper; let stand until hardened. Store in refrigerator if desired. Makes about 3 dozen cookies.

Drinks

Pineapple Energy Drink

   1 cup unsweetened pineapple juice
   ½ cup canned pineapple chunks
   2 heaping tbsp high protein powder
   2 tsp wheat germ oil
   honey to taste

Combine all ingredients in a blender and mix well. Chill before drinking.

Orange Julius

   1 cup milk
   3 ice cubes
   2 medium oranges
         or
   juice of 3 oranges if you don't
         like the pulp
   1 egg
   1 cup water
   ½ cup sugar (or more or less, to
         taste)

Dump it all in a blender and mix well.

Breads

Honey Date Walnut Bread

   1 cup water
   ¾ cup honey
   1 cup chopped dates
   1 egg
   2 tbsp wheat germ oil
   1½ cups stone ground whole wheat
         flour, unsifted
   ½ cup toasted wheat germ
   2 tbsp baking powder
   ⅔ tsp salt
   ½ cup chopped walnuts

Heat water to boiling. Add dates and cook for 3 minutes while stirring. Cool slightly. To wheat germ oil, gradually add honey and then the egg. Stir in date mixture and nuts. Add flour, wheat germ, baking powder and salt. Pour into greased 9" x 5" x 3" loaf pan. Bake at 300° for 1½ hours or until done. Cool on rack.

High Protein Bread

   1 pkg dry or 1 cake compressed
      yeast
   ¼ cup warm water
   1½ cups high protein powder
   3½ cups sifted flour
   1 tbsp salt
   ¼ cup sugar
   ⅓ cup soy flour
   ½ cup nonfat dry milk solids
   ¼ cup wheat germ
   1 tbsp melted shortening
   1⅓ cups water

Dissolve yeast in the warm water. Combine dry ingredients in mixing bowl. Add dissolved yeast, melted shortening and water, mixing to blend well. Knead dough until smooth and satiny. Place in well-greased bowl. Cover and let rise in warm place for 1½ hours. Shape into 2 loaves and place in greased pans. Cover and let stand about 55-60 minutes in warm place until dough fills the pans. Bake in pre-heated oven at 400° for 45 minutes.

High Protein Soft Gingerbread

1½ cups sifted high protein powder
¼ tsp baking soda
1½ tsp ginger
1½ tsp cinnamon
⅛ tsp cloves
¼ tsp salt
2 eggs
½ cup molasses
½ cup sour milk or buttermilk
⅓ cup butter or shortening
½ cup brown sugar

Pre-heat oven to 350°. Sift high protein powder, baking soda and spices into bowl; set aside. Put remaining ingredients into blender. Cover and process until blended. Pour into dry ingredients and mix well. Pour into greased 8" x 8" pan. Bake for 25 minutes.

Meat Dishes

Applesauce Meat Loaf

1½ pounds ground beef
1 egg, beaten
2 tbsp chopped onion
1 tsp allspice
1 cup applesauce
¼ cup high protein powder

Combine all ingredients. Pack into oiled loaf pan and bake for one hour at 350°.

Meat and Vegetable Burgers

1 pound ground round steak
1 cup ground raw carrots
1 cup ground raw potatoes
2 tbsp minced onion
2 tbsp minced parsley
⅓ cup toasted wheat germ
⅓ cup water, mixed with:
2 tbsp high protein powder
1 egg, slightly beaten

In a bowl, combine the ground meat, carrots, potatoes, onion, parsley, wheat germ and egg. Mix, add water and high protein, and then mix again thoroughly. Shape into patties and place on lightly oiled baking pan. Bake in a hot oven for 6 minutes on each side.

High Protein Croquettes

one 13 oz can of tuna fish
1 egg
¼ cup high protein powder
cheese, cut into 1 inch cubes
one 10 oz can cream of mushroom soup
¼ cup melted butter
1 tbsp minced parsley

Flake tuna and combine ingredients. Form balls around the cubes of cheese. Dip into wheat germ as breading and brown in hot oil.

Liver Loaf

1 pound liver: beef, pork, or lamb
1 cup high protein bread made into crumbs
1 medium sized onion
¼ cup chopped parsley
1 egg, slightly beaten
salt and pepper, to taste

Simmer liver gently in 1 cup boiling water for 10 minutes. Remove and grind liver and onion together in food chopper. Add bread crumbs, egg, water in which liver was cooked and seasonings. Mix well and put into a greased baking dish. Bake about 1 hour at 350°. Serve with mushroom sauce.

Mushroom Sauce

1 cup brown gravy
¼ tsp Worcestershire sauce
¼ tsp wheat germ oil
½ cup canned mushrooms

Combine all ingredients. Blend together and pour over liver loaf after heating sauce.

Desserts

Protein Mocha Frost

3 tbsp cocoa
3 tbsp sugar
2 heaping tbsp high protein powder
2/3 cup water
1 tbsp instant coffee
3 cups milk
1 pint ice cream
whipped cream - optional

In a saucepan, mix cocoa, sugar and high protein powder. Stir in water and cook the mixture about 3 minutes. Stir in coffee. Chill. When ready to serve, add milk and ice cream and beat in a mixer or blender until well mixed and frothy. Pour into tall glasses and garnish with whipped cream, if desired.

Holiday Health Roll

1 cup high protein powder
3/4 cup unsaturated peanut butter
1/2 cup honey
1/2 cup powdered milk
1 tbsp whole milk
1/3 cup chopped pineapple
1/3 cup chopped candied cherries
1/2 cup chopped pecans

Blend high protein powder, peanut butter and honey in mixing bowl. Mix powdered milk and whole milk together until a smooth paste is formed. Then knead in pineapple, cherries, pecans. Roll out onto waxed paper about 1½ inches in diameter and about 1 foot long. Roll up in waxed paper and place in refrigerator 3 to 4 hours. Slice and serve. Before wrapping health roll in waxed paper, it may be rolled in finely chopped nuts, or sunflower seeds, shredded coconut, raisins or any candied fruit may be added according to individual tastes.

TV Protein Snack

1 cup cottage cheese
1/2 cup plain yogurt

With electric blender, mix the ingredients together on low speed for 2 minutes. Place in a covered container and refrigerate. Good as a snack and delicious as a spread on toast.

Easy Pineapple Sticks

1 fresh pineapple
1/4 cup honey
1/2 cup sunflower seed meal
2 tbsp high protein powder

Prepare pineapple, slicing into sticks. Brush with honey. Place under medium broiler for approximately 2 minutes (using a cookie sheet). Mix seed with high protein powder and sprinkle over pineapple sticks.

Health Food Pudding

1 loaf oatmeal or high protein bread, made into crumbs
2 eggs
1¼ cubes safflower oil margarine
1/2 cup honey
1/2 cup raisins
1/2 cup chopped walnuts
1/4 cup half and half (light cream)
1/2 cup orange juice
1 small can fruit salad, drained
1 banana, 1 pear
1/2 cup high protein powder
1/2 cup wheat germ

Mix all ingredients together. Bake in a greased bread pan at 350° for 60 minutes or until brown crust forms.

High Protein Apple Crisp

    4 cups sliced cooking apples (quar-
        tered, cored and pared)
    1 tbsp lemon juice
    1/3 cup sifted high protein powder
    1/3 cup oats (uncooked)
    1/2 cup brown sugar
    1 tsp cinnamon
    1/4 cup melted (or soft) butter

Place apples in an oiled, shallow baking dish. Sprinkle lemon juice over the apples. Combine dry ingredients and then add melted butter, mixing until crumbly. Sprinkle crumb mixture over apples. Bake at 375° (pre-heated) for 30 minutes or until apples are tender. For added nourishment, sprinkle wheat germ on top before baking.

High Protein Peach Custard

    3/4 cup milk
    1/3 cup high protein powder
    1 tbsp honey
    1/3 cup canned peaches, drained
    1 egg

Place all ingredients, except the egg, in a blender. When ingredients are well mixed, add the egg and blend for 3 seconds. Pour into 3 greased four ounce custard pans. Put into pan of hot water and bake at 325° for 20 minutes.

Breakfast Cereal

Granola

    5 cups oats
    5 cups graham flour
    1 cup corn meal
    1/2 cup rye flour
    1/2 cup flaked coconut
    3/4 cup brown sugar
    1/2 cup almonds (optional)
    1/4-1/2 cup wheat germ
    1 tbsp salt
    1/2 cup salad oil
    1/2 cup honey
    3/4 cup water

Mix dry ingredients well. Sprinkle on oil while stirring, then honey and then water. Spread on 2 cookie sheets and bake at 300° for 45 minutes; stir every 15 minutes. Let stand in turned off oven until cool.

SECTION VII

CLINICS

1

On Conducting Coaching Clinics

The year 1972 will go down in weightlifting history as the year weightlifting clinics began to emerge on a large scale. Such clinics began with the annual Teen-Age Camp for the National Teen-Age Champions in 1966. Then in 1972 a clinic at the Nationals and ten Christmas clinics were added to this annual Teen-Age Camp. The prospects for future clinics look very good. Easter clinics are planned, and the Regional Championships have been designated as the prime time to hold clinics. Already results are being felt. Technical information from just these beginnings has spread all over the United States. Lifters on one side of the country are finding out what lifters on the other side of the country are doing. Most important, the vast technical knowledge across the nation is reaching young lifters. These lifters will no longer have to spend many years of trial and error learning how to lift and how to train.

The clinics vary widely in length from a few hours to a couple of weeks. This means that various lengths of programs have to be planned. But whether the clinic is short or long, the main thrust at these clinics in the immediate future should be the teaching of how to plan a long range routine and the teaching of proper technique. At the previous clinics, it has been found that even the young lifters have some knowledge of individual aspects of the lifts. What they do not understand is how to organize this knowledge into individualized cohesive one or two year plans which show each lifter how to progress over a long time span.

At such a clinic, several factors of planning a long range routine should be included: (1) Cycling of Intensity, (2) Cycling of Load, (3) Flexibility Work, and (4) Conditioning Work. This is because continued progress in weightlifting depends greatly on how intensely a lifter lifts at various times, how long he lifts at various times, how flexible he is, and what type of general physical condition he is in. There are many fine points of lifting which can be taught (such as special routines, special assistant exercises, special meet preparations, and nutrition), all very important in themselves but all of which need to fit into the general framework of long range planning in order to have any real meaning. These aspects of lifting and others should be considered, at least in the near future, only when the first four factors listed above have been covered at the clinic.

Technique is believed best taught at clinics by one person, or else various phases of a technique can be taught by different persons, each responsible for a certain aspect of the technique. This manner of teaching technique has been borrowed successfully from clinics in other sports. The idea is to not present conflicting views by the coaches at one clinic. This is not to say that there is no justification for diversity. Undoubtedly a lifter or coach can learn certain things from one clinic, and he can learn other things by attending another clinic. In this way he can make comparisons. But in other sports it has been found that teaching various techniques at the same clinic produces confusion instead of learning.

A very important outcome of a clinic should be enthusiasm. However, the teaching of technical material will not alone impart enthusiasm. Communication between the coaching staff and the students should be very open if this enthusiasm is to result from the clinic. This is why it is strongly recommended that many times during the formal presentation of technical material, "rap" or "bull" sessions should be held. Many ideas emerge at these sessions, and they are invaluable to promoting the kind of rapport that is necessary between coach and lifter.

In order to run a successful clinic as discussed above, the groundwork must be laid far in advance to create favorable conditions. This is where organization and good public relations are necessary. First, a coaching staff for the clinic should be chosen and a site obtained. At previous clinics, colleges, YMCAs, Boys' Clubs and military bases have been the most cooperative in lending or renting the use of their facilities. To keep the expenses down on the facilities, local clubs such as Kiwanis, Lions and Jaycees can be asked to sponsor all or part of the cost. Another idea is to volunteer to exchange services with the people of the facility which is being used. For example, in return for the use of a YMCA's facilities, a certain number of classes in weightlifting could be conducted for interested members.

When the coaches to run the clinic are being chosen, it is recommended that one be chosen as head coach. That is, one person is chosen who will be the boss and has the last say, after consultation with the other coaches, on what the plan of action will be. This is the method used in clinics in other sports, and it has worked the best in past weightlifting clinics. This is not to say that the head coach is the only person who has any say in what goes on during the clinic. If he is a good head coach, he will get together with his assistants, present to them his plan and then work with them in formulating how the plan can best be presented. Close rapport between the head coach and assistants is a must. The coaching staff should be chosen with this in mind so that this rapport stands the best possible chance of developing.

Once the coaches and site have been chosen, an information flyer should be sent not only to the Regional Chairman but also to other key weightlifting personnel who are active in the area. This should be done two to three months in advance of the clinic. The flyer should include who the coaches will be, what will be covered at the clinic, what it will cost, what supplies will be needed at the clinic, how long the clinic is to be, what transportation is available, and any items which might be peculiar to the particular clinic being held.

Next in organization should be the planning of equipment for the best efficiency. It has been found that one platform with one Olympic bar per six lifters is the bare minimum. It would be better to have only four lifters per platform. It has also been found that it is difficult to give adequate coaching attention to many lifters at one time. Therefore, it is recommended that one coach be in charge of each platform, with perhaps the head coach supervising the whole operation. When other pieces of equipment are needed, the maximum ratio should again be six to one and preferably four to one.

Of final importance in organization is the planning for the presentation of the clinic. Whether the clinic is long or short, a schedule of what is to be presented at what time should be handed out to all the assistant coaches and the lifters and coaches who attend. This gives direction to the clinic, shows the people participating what material is scheduled to be covered and, in general, gives an air of professionalism. This promotes confidence in the clinic right from the beginning. In addition, along with a schedule, mimeographed copies of major points to be covered at the clinic should be handed out. A clinic is so short, whether it lasts a few hours or a couple of weeks, that unless major points are given out in writing, much of the material will be forgotten. This happens in spite of the fact that the participants take notes. It has been found that a clinic goes all too fast and that it is just not possible for the participant to fully retain all that is taught without some written material which he can look at again once the clinic is over.

There are some miscellaneous things which can be done to make a clinic more successful. One is to arrange to have a video tape machine at the clinic so that the lifters can immediately see themselves lifting, and technique can be quickly analyzed. A local service club might donate the funds to rent such a machine for the duration of the clinic, if one is not available. The local AAU may have one which is at the disposal of AAU sports teams in its area. If a video tape machine is not available, then the lifter can be filmed. This can be done at the beginning of a long camp so that the films can be developed and on hand in time to show at the end of the camp. If the camp is short, then an analysis by the coaches of the filming can be sent with the film to the lifter. One roll of film per lifter would then be used.

Another thing to make a clinic more successful would be to check to see if a top American lifter who is articulate is available; if he is, then it would be well worthwhile to invite him to speak. He can greatly add to the enthusiasm of the camp, and he will have good insights. These insights will be a help to the coaching staff as well as the participants because this is one way coaches stay abreast of new things being tried.

A third thing to add to a clinic's success is to give some little souvenir from the camp to the participants; this would be a lasting symbol of the clinic for each to take home. They are each going to take away a lot of knowledge, but some little thing such as a tee shirt with the clinic title on it can be a nice memento.

Finally, under the category of public relations, there should be proper publicity in the town before the clinic gets under way. This involves the people who are furnishing the facilities, the press (newspaper, tv, radio), local stores, and local coaches and athletic organizations. There should appear an announcement of the camp and a picture. Local coaches should be invited to observe some of the sessions along with their athletes. Even if few come, much will have been done for public relations. Most important of all, the local community will know that in the sport of weightlifting something is happening. People will join and people will contribute to something they think is active, and weightlifting needs to give that impression. Then, following the clinic there should be a release to the press as to what happened, along with some pictures.

There is more that can be said about putting on clinics, but to say more would probably be to get into specifics that can best be dealt with at the local level. What was said here was to offer a general guide. It is hoped that this guide will be of service, not necessarily for following it to the letter but in showing what has been done successfully. It will be improved upon as the American experience with weightlifting clinics begins to accumulate. For this to happen, weightlifting needs you, the AAU official, you, the coach, and you, the experienced lifter to hold clinics. Hold them for advanced lifters and hold them for beginning lifters. We not only need to teach more technical information, but also we need desperately to increase by one hundred fold the number of new lifters in the United States. The champion teams of other countries were built by teaching sound technical information to masses of lifters. From the masses emerged the champions. The clinic is a perfect way to gather new people into lifting. Hold hour long clinics for such groups as boys at the local playground, the local YMCA, the Boys' Club, and the football, track, wrestling and gymnastic coaches. Then the next time, hold a longer one. You will see your base of lifters and your base of outside help grow. Your technical knowledge will then reach more people, and from an increase in numbers will come the talented lifters who will someday challenge the best in the world.

Junior Olympic Training Camp Schedule
Monday, July 21 to Saturday, July 26

This is included in this book as an example of a training camp schedule.

Monday

7:30 a.m.	Breakfast
9:30-11:30 a.m.	Train with weights (coaching staff)
	1. snatch style
	2. snatch assistant exercises
12:00-1:30 p.m.	Lunch
2:00-4:00 p.m.	Train with weights (coaching staff)
	1. clean style
	2. clean assistant exercises
4:30-6:00 p.m.	Style Analysis - films, etc. (coaching staff)
6:00-7:00 p.m.	Dinner
7:00-8:30 p.m.	Training Plan (Miller)
11:00 p.m.	Bed

Tuesday

7:30 a.m.	Breakfast
9:30-11:30 a.m.	Train with weights (coaching staff)
	1. jerk style
	2. jerk assistant exercises
12:00-1:30 p.m.	Lunch
2:00-4:00 p.m.	Train with weights (coaching staff)
	1. clean and jerk style
	2. remedial exercises
4:30-6:00 p.m.	Training Plan (Miller)
6:00-7:00 p.m.	Dinner
7:00-8:30 p.m.	Style Analysis (Mills)
11:00 p.m.	Bed

Wednesday

7:30 a.m.	Breakfast
9:30-11:30 a.m.	Train with weights (coaching staff)
	1. snatch style
	2. snatch assistant exercises
12:00-1:30 p.m.	Lunch
2:00-4:00 p.m.	Training with weights (coaching staff)
	1. clean and jerk style
	2. leg training
4:30-6:00 p.m.	Training Plan (Miller)
6:00-7:00 p.m.	Dinner
7:00 p.m.	Typical New England Entertainment
11:00 p.m.	Bed

Thursday

7:30 a.m.	Breakfast
9:30-11:30 a.m.	Train with weights (coaching staff)
	1. clean and jerk style
	2. snatch style

Thursday (cont.)

12:00-1:30 p.m.	Lunch
2:00-4:00 p.m.	Games related to lifting (coaching staff)
	1. soccer
	2. volleyball
	3. high jump and broad jump
4:30-6:00 p.m.	Style Analysis (Mills)
6:00-7:00 p.m.	Dinner
7:00-8:30 p.m.	Backstage Strategy and Meet Preparation (Mills)
11:00 p.m.	Bed

Friday

7:30 a.m.	Breakfast
9:30-11:30 a.m.	Train with weights (coaching staff)
	1. snatch style
	2. clean style
12:00-1:30 p.m.	Lunch
2:00-4:00 p.m.	Train with weights (coaching staff)
	1. readaptability training
	2. functional readiness
4:30-6:00 p.m.	Prevention and Care of Athletic Injuries (Cameron)
6:00-7:00 p.m.	Dinner
7:00-8:30 p.m.	Peaking (coaching staff)
8:30 p.m.-?	Typical New England Entertainment

Saturday

break camp and on to new lifting horizons!

Coaching Staff

1. Carl Miller
2. Joe Mills
3. John Coleman
4. Joe Caron
5. Denis Reno
6. Frank Clark
7. Jim Decoste
8. Mark Cameron
9. Frank Gancarz

SECTION VIII

INTERNATIONAL TRIP PREPARATIONS

Introduction

After this introduction will appear some letters I sent concerning some of our international trips between 1973 and 1975. These were very successful trips marked by a high success ratio of attempts made, personal records broken, high team spirit and team cohesiveness. These letters will give coaches, athletes and officials some idea of the thinking behind these successful trips. There is a great body of knowledge to be put down in writing about this subject in the future.

The basis for a successful trip revolves around sincere communication. For example, I wrote to some lifters seven times before training camp. With such communication, many things such as starting poundages and jumps never became a problem because of complete understanding. Getting across, for example, the idea of being flexible in this area of starting poundages and jumps needs this communication. With one lifter, I pointed out fifteen alternative strategies for the first attempt and the succeeding jumps. He had never thought of the various alternatives.

Successful international teams and trips do not just happen. The execution of a successful trip should come off like "no big deal" and should just flow. However, what goes into the many facets of a trip from selecting an international match to its completion involves much thought, philosophy and organization, and it involves hours and hours of work to make it happen.

2

Letters Concerning Some International Trips

To: Leading Candidates for United States Summer Weightlifting Team Tour of Europe

From: Carl Miller, Head Coach

Congratulations on being selected as a leading candidate for the Europe Tour. I know you have just received a letter from our team manager, Denis Reno. Now I am looking forward to hearing from you. This is a big moment for you, in particular, and for United States weightlifting in general. Many people have worked hard to make such a trip possible, and now it is up to us to make the trip a success. If you make the final selection and are chosen to make the trip, you should know the following information.

The demands on your physical, mental and emotional energies will be great. You will be competing 4 times within 16 days. Back in 1958 the Russians came to the United States and had 3 matches with the United States in a comparable time. Those Russian athletes who prepared themselves well after the tryouts and disciplined themselves during the duration of the grueling match schedule held up superbly. We know this is your goal, and we want to do everything possible to help you reach it. This is why, as head coach, I am making some statements and recommendations and asking you some questions.

Take everything you will need with you. Don't assume you will be able to get anything when you are there. And make sure your belt measures $3\frac{7}{8}$ inches in width before you leave the United States. Find enclosed a brief summary of the rules and note especially those concerning tape on the thumb and other wraps.

Measure your grip on the bar for both the snatch and the clean and jerk. And take care of those calluses. Keep them trim with emery cloth and soft with lotion.

Practice lifting in different surroundings and at different times. Practice using different lengths of warm-up times. Practice different jumps in weights. Part of the purpose of this trip is to get you mentally tough for what we hope will be bigger competition for you later on. And this involves lifting in all types of conditions.

We all have a lot of work ahead of us. While every attempt will be made to consider your individual differences, we expect full team cooperation. Be on time and look sharp. A positive mental attitude is a must. In this, your first international trip abroad, for your development it is imperative to total. Your successful performance both as an individual and as part of the United States team will greatly inspire you, other lifters, coaches and officials to continue our program toward reaching the top in international weightlifting competition.

On the following pages are questions I would like you to answer and mail back to me so that I can have everything organized for the trip. This will include talking with you many times during our camp over relevant matters. Some questions you may have already answered in response to Denis Reno's letter. You needn't answer them twice. We are interested in you doing your best, so please answer the questions as accurately as you can. If there is anything we can do between now and when we leave, please let us know.

Looking forward to seeing you at the Seniors,

Carl Miller

Athlete's Information Sheet

Name _____ Weight Class _____ Phone _____

Address _____ City _____ State _____

Age _____ Birthday _____

1. Training Bodyweight _____

2. Last Three Competitions

    #1
    Bodyweight _____ Competition Date _____ Competition Name _____

        Attempts
                Snatch _____ _____ _____   Best Lift _____

                C & J _____ _____ _____   Best Lift _____

                                                  Total _____

    #2
    Bodyweight _____ Competition Date _____ Competition Name _____

        Attempts
                Snatch _____ _____ _____   Best Lift _____

                C & J _____ _____ _____   Best Lift _____

                                                  Total _____

    #3
    Bodyweight _____ Competition Date _____ Competition Name _____

        Attempts
                Snatch _____ _____ _____   Best Lift _____

                C & J _____ _____ _____   Best Lift _____

                                                  Total _____

3. How did you plan, and what plan did you use for your last three competitions?

4. What is your plan for this competition?

5. What is your warm-up schedule for the snatch and for the clean and jerk? (Please list time needed.)

6. What type of atmosphere do you like around you when preparing to lift (e.g. quiet determination, pep talks)? Name specifics.

7. Are there any special foods or drinks you will require during the competition? Before or after? (Remember that when in doubt, lift with a hungry feeling; you don't want to lift with food putrifying in your stomach either because too much has been eaten or because it is food that is hard to digest, such as French fries, malts, steaks, any meat, cheese and eggs.)

8. Are there any special things we should know in order to help you be the best prepared possible?

To: Members of International Selection Committee
From: Carl Miller, Head Coach of Under 23 Trip to Europe
Subject: European Trip

In a separate report, which you will receive from team manager Denis Reno, are the statistics of our matches in Europe. First, you will notice that all four of the matches were won. Beyond this are many positive noteworthy aspects. 1) There were no bombouts. 2) We had better than a two thirds success rate. (This is very noteworthy since it was the first international competition for all but one of these young men and the first competition abroad for all.) 3) Our best lifting took place in the last meets even though we started out good. Both the second and third points lend credence to the idea that initial success leads to further success with heavier weights (rather than leading to low totals).

From the very moment these matches were set up, Denis Reno and I contacted the prospective lifters and expounded on the priorities. This contact took place by mail, at meets and at clinics. These priorities were, in order: 1) to total, 2) to win, and 3) to make records.

My travels in going to meets and putting on clinics (actually started before the National Coaching Plan became a reality) made it possible to have a real working knowledge of individual lifters' performances on and off the platform. This inspired trust on both parts, mine and the athletes'.

The week long camp held prior to leaving for Europe was invaluable in cementing this above-mentioned trust and also in building team cohesiveness. In all types of team performance, a respect for each other's personalities and ways of doing things is a must. As long as the one goal of lifting the best possible was observed, personality differences could not only be respected but could also be drawn upon for team strength. This training camp, combined with prior personal contact with the lifters, plus the careful up-to-date records kept by Denis Reno over a period of 6 months, made this group of individuals a "team" before we even left for Europe.

This openness and trust was evident after the first match with Germany. There were aspects that both the athletes and coaches wanted ironed out to make the rest of the trip even more productive. This was done in a successful manner as witnessed by the even better performances which resulted as the tour continued.

A theme constantly stressed at the camp and during the trip was to keep everything positive. This was especially pinpointed with style. Final preparation for lifting in international competition was needed to reinforce everything positive each lifter does within his style to make him lift more. This is not to say that realities were masked over; lifters and coaches were all cognizant of major style flaws, but to try to change them at this point would have led to confusion and sub-par performance. So a "polishing" of styles took place. There was one notable exception to this, and it occurred during our longest break, between the Spain and England matches. Even then we were trying to interject only one change to get a better performance, and it worked. When all the matches were over, then I talked with the lifters individually and gave them our recommendations on how to improve their performances through style and training modifications. This was the time that was appropriate both from the success point of view of this tour and the receptiveness of the athletes.

As was stated above, the lifting performances started out well. The reason they got better was not only because of great desire and team spirit, but also because of the international experience. After the match with France, a French official told me that they had thought the match, because it lined up close on paper, would go to the French because they had much more international experience and thus would stand up under pressure better. My answer to him was that these young men had positive attitudes when they came overseas, and they had one successful international match under their belt (Germany). As time went on and they had more international experience, they became even better. I cannot stress this experience enough. The European lifter gets so much international experience that he develops faster. That is one reason why they lift so much at a young age. What they get in a year, many of our lifters will not get in four. And in our country where one faces hardships in training after finishing school, experience such as this is even more important to our lifters than it is to their European counterparts for whom these hardships, in many cases, are greatly eased.

This international experience is not only important from the individual standpoint but also from the team standpoint. In England they said it was the best performance they had seen by a U.S. team technique-wise and team spirit-wise in many, many years. This was at the end of the tour. In the middle lifting session of that last match, for example, our lifters made 16 out of 18 attempts with 4 personal records. It could be taken for granted that our technique would be good since we have been having extensive clinics for the past almost two years, but what is even more significant is that the technique was so good at the last match and that the spirit was at its best even though it had started out high in Germany. This is important because after being together for so long a team either pulls together to better performances or pulls apart and sinks. I believe that the technique being so good at the end of the tour was a result of team spirit, of everyone pulling for each individual both on and off the platform. The lifters wanted to improve, and they did so propped up by the security of the team encouragement.

The positive performances by this team were a result of ability, desire and determination of the official, coaches and athletes who were on the trip. They were also a result of the positive programs instituted by the National Weightlifting Committee. All the things which have been worked for by so many people had a positive result. Indeed, this was a big positive result because not only were we competing against individual lifters, but we were also up against National Coaching Plans of other countries which have full-time paid National Coaches. These plans have been in operation for a much longer time than ours (in the case of France, since 1966). While this trip was a success, we all realize it should be viewed as something to build upon because we have a long way to go to become competitive with the Eastern Europeans. Nevertheless, performances of this kind resulting from our beginnings can only inspire us all to continue with even greater determination.

Respectfully submitted,

Carl Miller
Head Coach, 1974 Under 23 Europe Tour

P.S. Based on his performance on this trip, on behalf of the coaches I would like to recommend Lee James, 181 lb. class, to be a member of the International Team that goes to Manila. His performance of 308-374 was a marked increase over his best at the Seniors, which in turn was a marked increase over his last previous performance. His betterment of style on the tour is also noteworthy. This and his extreme dedication are the type of things for which we want to reward our lifters in order for them to improve and to show an example to other aspiring lifters.

Dear   ,

Congratulations on being selected for the World Youth Games which are to be held July 5-12 in Marseille, France. You will be receiving more information and details from Manager Marty Cypher. I can tell you now that there will be one class lifting each day, starting July 5th with the flyweight class. We will be meeting at York College on Thursday, June 26th for a training camp. We will leave York College on Thursday, July 2nd and return the 14th of July. The first thing you should do is get yourself a passport, now! This takes about 4-6 weeks to get processed.

Our youth competition last summer in Europe was very successful, and we want to build on this. Let me orient you to some things that we feel are important.

Priorities - The first priority is to total, the second is to place as high as possible, and the third is to make personal records. It is very important to remember these priorities; this is how sound success is built.

Team Spirit - Among the lifters there will be many different types of personalities. None is better than any other, just different. Let your personalities mesh, not clash. Take strength in the diversity that you will find, and you will all pull together. Remember the one goal - team success - at all times, and this will be easy. Part of having team spirit is to act the part of who you are - a champion. That includes looking neat and sharp. You are representing not only yourself, but also your neighborhood, your city, your state, and the United States of America.

Training Until Competition - Probably the greatest problem you will have will be overtraining. If you have any problems with training routines before coming to the camp, please write me. Let us not have anybody come to camp overtrained, drained because he had an overabundance of enthusiasm and did not use his head and plan well. By the same token, don't just lay off. You have all heard about the lifter who just goes to bed before competition and then wonders why he doesn't lift well. Make your habits, training and day to day living as normal as possible.

Prevention - There are a few things that should be taken care of to prevent little but important things from going wrong before competition. One is to take care of calluses. Another is to take extra precautions against colds. Take some extra vitamins, and make sure you eat a balanced diet and get normal rest. Torn calluses or colds can undo all the training you have done. Speaking about vitamins, you may want to take some extra vitamin C and electrolytes (see enclosure). If you want to discuss this further, please write.

Experimentation - This is not the time for experimenting and great changes. You want to train as normally for this meet as you would for any other big meet. This goes for style too; don't be changing your style even though it is not perfect. Polish up what you have. However, there are some things that aren't drastic changes which you might want to work with since you have sufficient time to try them out. One, try going on a high carbohydrate diet for two to three days and note your energy level during this time. I mean instead of a lot of protein and fat, substitute such things as spaghetti, macaroni, rice, cereals, bread, fruits and vegetables. This is not good as a steady diet, but it can give you much extra energy before a competition if eaten for two to three days prior to it. Experimentation with this once or twice will let you know whether or not you want to use it for your competition.

There are two things to experiment with in order to get used to using them. One, take alternating hot and cold showers after a workout. This has been proven to lead to faster and more complete recovery from a workout. Take a hot shower for a-

136

bout a minute followed by cold for 15 seconds; repeat three or four times, ending up with a cold shower. Two, get used to a sauna. Don't stay in it to get drained, but use it once or twice a week just to get used to it. Then if you have to use it to lose weight, your body will have been used to it and it won't come as a shock. Under no circumstances take diuretics to lose weight.

Equipment - Take everything you need. Don't expect to buy what you need in France, although you might be able to; come prepared. Remember that your shoes should have no flanges, and your belt should be $3\frac{7}{8}$ inches wide. Most belts sold in the United States are 4 inches, so have them shaved. If there is any new equipment you need to get, do it now and get used to it, not at training camp or in France.

Drugs - I am assuming that no one takes hard or soft drugs. Have absolutely nothing in your possession, or you could very well wind up in jail for a long time, besides embarrassing the team and your country.

Relaxation - I don't mean to treat each of the following as equal in importance; I am just mentioning them to bring them to mind. If you are a religious person, continue your practice. A tremendous peace of mind can be gained. If you have gone into meditation or hypnosis, then continue. There will be times you will have time on your hands. If you are a reader, read, and don't forget to bring reading material along. You won't be busy every minute, and you will want something to relax you.

These are just a few things that we feel are important. Please feel free to contact me or any of the other coaches. We want you to perform your best. Good luck, and we will be looking forward to hearing from you before camp or seeing you at camp.

Sincerely,

Carl Miller
Head Coach, Under 20 Youth Team

P.S. One final note: Everybody, on his day of lifting, will lift at 6:00 p.m. Do your training at this time to get used to lifting at this hour. Also, weigh yourself at 4:45 p.m.; it does make a difference. I don't know the type of auditorium you will be lifting in, so practice lifting in different surroundings. And practice using different lengths of warm-up times and different jumps in weights. Part of the purpose of this trip is to get you mentally tough for what we hope will be bigger competitions for you later on, and this involves lifting in all types of conditions.

Below are listed some lifters of the world who total near you or above you (there are also many, many others who total below you). While this is realistic and may disturb some of you who are used to having no competition, remember a few things. Some of these lifters may not be in France for a variety of reasons such as past the age limit, too far to come, or injuries. American teams in many sports (a good example is gymnastics) have good talent but never progress to their potential because of lack of international experience. You need this type of competition to bring out the best in you both now and in the future. You are a developmental team. We certainly don't feel this is an "end all competition". You were chosen for your present ability and your potential for the future. Right now some foreign lifters are lifting heavier weights earlier in life than we are. With the program we are building, we feel you will catch them in the future and you will beat many of them now. You wouldn't have been chosen nor would all the money have been spent and the time and effort have been made by countless numbers of people if we didn't have confidence in you. Remember the priorities for progress: 1) total, 2) place as high as possible, and 3) go after personal records. If you follow these, you will have a successful competition. You are representing yourself, your family, your neighborhood, your city, your state and your country, and we are sure everybody will be proud of you when you return.

114

Danilchenko	USSR	440	187-253
Chiru	Rum	429	192-237
Seweryn	Pol	419	176-231
Adamczyk	Pol	409	
Cachon	Spain	396	171-225
Mehner	DDR	380	159-220
Torriko	Swed	375	
MERAZ	USA	363	154-209
Walk	DDR	357	
Eschnessy	W.Ger	357	
Obermuller	W.Ger	357	

123

Weres	Rum	462	209-253
Dimitrov	Bul	451	198-253
Zajdel	Pol	446	
Valle	Spain	434	187-247
Lenartowicz	Pol	423	181-242
Buhleier	Pol	423	
Lipinski	DDR	418	
Mavius	DDR	418	
KESSLER	USA	413	

132

Dembonchik	Pol	539	242-297
Buta	Rum	511	220-292
Pawluk	Pol	506	220-286
Szarnuewicz	Pol	501	225-275
Rutter	Czek	501	214-286
Kunchev	Bul	496	209-286
Casado	Spain	491	220-270
Janke	DDR	473	
WARNER	USA	468	204-264
SCHAKE	USA	445	200-245

148

Belkov	Bul	582	264-319
Neguer	W.Ger	582	
COHEN	USA	556	242-314
Sygnowski	Pol	556	248-308
			253-303
Palos	Rum	556	259-297
Kurarkov	Pol	556	
Horschig	DDR	550	
Schliwka	DDR	545	225-319
Ambrass	DDR	535	
Wollman	W.Ger	535	

165

Totamish	USSR	671	286-385
Mitkov	Bul	665	292-375
			(386)
Groh	W.Ger	627	
Bergmann	W.Ger	594	
Pryzbtkiski	Pol	594	
Szymanski	Pol	594	264-330

181

Appel	W.Ger	660	
Mils	Pol	649	
Belikhousky	Bul	649	286-363
Herr	W.Ger	635	
LUJAN	USA	628	275-353
Jazlowiecki	Pol	628	264-353
			286-341

165 (cont.)					181 (cont.)			
Karlson	Swed	577			Stepak	USSR	616	275-341
MUCARDO	USA	572	248-325					
JULIUS	USA	572	253-319					
Kongehl	DDR	565						

198			
Leuko	USSR	678	303-375
Turczak	Pol	661	286-375
Chizhov	USSR	655	292-363
Meinecke	DDR	661	
Walo	DDR	655	
CLARK	USA	617	270-347
Daub	W.Ger	617	

Looking forward to seeing you soon with great expectations,

Carl Miller, Head Coach

Marty Cypher, Manager
Dick "Smitty" Smith, Asst. Coach
Howard Cohen, Asst. Coach
Butch Toth, Asst. Coach

Marty,

Please find below a schedule for our camp. I will arrive Wednesday the 25th around 5:30 PM into Baltimore. You said we leave Monday afternoon for France. Since we want everybody in Thursday the 26th in the PM, would you send out to the lifters and coaches when they should be there (Thursday PM the 26th), what airports to go into, and how to get to York College. Ask for their flight schedules so in case we can get transportation out there (to the airport), we can meet them. You might duplicate this schedule so they have an idea of what to expect at the camp.

Thursday 26th	Friday 27th	Saturday 28th
Lunch	Breakfast	Breakfast
Check in at York College	White House Special Tour	Individual discussions with
4:45 PM Weigh-in	Lunch (big)	coaches by lifters
5:00 PM Dinner	Rest	Lunch
6:30 PM Orientation	4:45 PM Weigh-in	Weightlifting Tape -
	5:00 PM Dinner (light)	psychological
	6:00 PM Train	Weightlifting Movie - style
	1) practice 15 lb jumps	Group Discussion with coaches
	2) practice 9 min waits	4:45 PM Weigh-in
		Dinner
		Entertainment

Sunday 29th	Monday 30th
Breakfast	Breakfast
Church or Rest	Any needed discussion
12:45 PM Weigh-in	Orientation to France - people, customs, etc.
Lunch (light)	Rest
2:00 PM Train	Lunch
1) practice 25 lb jumps	Finish Packing
2) practice 12 min rest	Leave for airport!
Dinner	
Psychological Movie	
Group Discussion with coaches	

I know this may have to be changed, but people, especially young keyed-up ones, need some stability to calm them down. This schedule will help. We will go over training when they get there; this will be largely what they already have programmed based on what we have talked about with them before. Even though they are individually programmed and some may work out only once, I want everybody to go through warm-ups together. Any advice or suggestions on your part or on the parts of the other coaches are welcome.

See you soon,

Carl

cc: Cohen, Smitty, Toth

www.ingramcontent.com/pod-product-compliance
Lightning Source LLC
Chambersburg PA
CBHW080404270326
41927CB00015B/3342

* 9 7 8 1 6 3 2 9 3 2 1 8 1 *